Oncology

Oxford Core Texts

Clinical Dermatology

Clinical Skills

Endocrinology

Health and Illness in the Community

Human Physiology

Medical Genetics

Medical Imaging

Neurology

Oncology

Palliative Care

Psychiatry

Oncology

SECOND EDITION

Dr Max Watson BD, MRCGP, MSc
Honorary Consultant in Palliative Medicine, The Princess Alice Hospice, Esher
Research Fellow, Belfast City Hospital

Professor Ann Barrett MD, FRCR, FRCP, FMedSci
Professor of Oncology, University of East Anglia
Honorary Consultant in Clinical Oncology, Norfolk and Norwich University Hospital
Previously, Professor of Clinical Oncology, University of Glasgow

Professor Roy AJ Spence OBE, MA, MD, FRCS
Consultant Surgeon, Belfast City Hospital
Honorary Professor, Queen's University, Belfast
Honorary Professor, University of Ulster

Professor Chris Twelves BMedSci, FRCP (London & Glasgow), MD
Professor of Clinical Cancer Pharmacology, University of Leeds
Honorary Consultant in Medical Oncology, Bradford NHS Hospital Foundation Trust and Leeds Teaching Hospitals

Dr Mary Drake *Consultant Haematologist, Belfast City Hospital* contributed the chapter on haematological malignancies

Dr Paula Scullin *Specialist Registrar Oncology Department, Belfast City Hospital* and **Dr Max Watson** edited the associated web pages at
http://www.oxfordtextbooks.co.uk/orc/watson

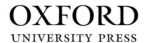

OXFORD
UNIVERSITY PRESS

OXFORD
UNIVERSITY PRESS

Great Clarendon Street, Oxford OX2 6DP

Oxford University Press is a department of the University of Oxford.
It furthers the University's objective of excellence in research, scholarship,
and education by publishing worldwide in

Oxford New York

Athens Auckland Bangkok Bogotá Buenos Aires Calcutta
Cape Town Chennai Dar es Salaam Delhi Florence Hong Kong Istanbul
Karachi Kuala Lumpur Madrid Melbourne Mexico City Mumbai
Nairobi Paris São Paulo Singapore Taipei Tokyo Toronto Warsaw

with associated companies in Berlin Ibadan

Oxford is a registered trade mark of Oxford University Press
in the UK and in certain other countries

Published in the United States
by Oxford University Press Inc., New York

© Oxford University Press, 2006

British Library Cataloguing in Publication Data

Data available

Library of Congress Cataloguing in Publication Data

ISBN 0 19 856757 X   978 0 19 856757 8

10 9 8 7 6 5 4 3 2 1

Typeset by EXPO Holdings Sdn Bhd, Malaysia
Printed in Great Britain
on acid-free paper by
Ashford Colour Press Ltd, Gosport, Hampshire

Preface

The aim of the second edition of this core text is to provide a compact, easy to read overview of modern adult oncology, suitable for students completing their undergraduate oncology attachments or junior doctors and nurses beginning work on oncology or haematology wards.

In support of this aim the size of the text has been reduced to allow the reader to grasp the essentials of the subject quickly. Special attention has been paid to the rapid changes in oncology which are beginning to have a major impact on current treatments. The first chapters deal with the concepts behind modern cancer treatment and the remainder are concerned with outlining the background and management of the common UK malignancies.

By use of highlighted text boxes readers are introduced to 'Key Facts' and 'Future Possibilities' in cancer management. The 'Stop and Think' and 'Test Yourself' text boxes encourage the reader not only to check their grasp of the topic but also grapple with some of the ethical challenges of current oncological practice.

The book has been written by clinical specialists from the five main cancer treatment areas, including medical and clinical oncology, surgery, haematology, and palliative medicine, and is thus centred on practical and current clinical practice.

http://www.oxfordtextbooks.co.uk/orc/watson/
The use of a dedicated web site with the book allows readers to benefit from well-illustrated common clinical scenarios, without the expense of a full colour text book. The site is divided into five different areas concerned with the clinical management of patients with lung, breast, bowel, prostate, and ovarian tumours. Through the site students can follow the clinical journey of a patient with one of these common cancers and have the chance to view X-rays, scans, blood films, etc. At the end of each web chapter there is a short MCQ assessment based on the book, allowing self-assessment. With the advantage of a dedicated web site as a teaching resource we hope the book will also prove to be a useful tool for those involved in undergraduate teaching.

As we have written and edited this text we have been once again reminded not only of the scope, promise, and rapid scientific development but also of increasing patient-centred compassion in modern UK oncology. We hope that readers of the core text will be as enthused, challenged, and encouraged by these developments as we have been in producing it.

M.W.
A.B.
R.S.
C.T.

Acknowledgements

The authors are pleased to acknowledge the great help received from Oxford University Press, and in particular from Anna Read, Colin McDougal, Ruth Craven, and Caroline Connolly through the long gestation period of this second edition.

No textbook 'is an island' and we must individually acknowledge the work of those involved in completing the first edition and thank them for allowing us to use and update their material: Peter Adamson, Brew Atkinson, Ronnie Atkinson, Patrick Bell, Robin Davidson, Ruth Eakin, Paul Harkin, David Harmon, Paddy Johnston, Patrick Keane, Frank Kee, John Kelly, Sheila Kelly, Richard Kennedy, Michael Lee, Seamus McAleer, Ultan McDermott, Sarah McKenna, Damian McManus, Kieran McManus, Curly Morris, William Odling-Smee, Brian Orr, Angus Patterson, John Price, Hilary Russell, Frank Sullivan, William Torreggiani, and Bridgette Widemann.

We are also grateful to those who have helped in the provision of illustrations, photographs, and radiological images.

The drive behind this text has come from the questions and interest of medical students whose enthusiasm to learn makes teaching and writing worthwhile.

We must also acknowledge the input and comments of colleagues who have reviewed the text during its formation. Their willingness to help and share their expertise so freely has been greatly appreciated. The ensuing discussions have been invaluable.

Finally we wish to acknowledge the support and understanding of our respective families, for whom this book has been yet another incursion into family life.

M.W
A.B.
R.S.
C.T.

Foreword

Cancer encompasses a diverse range of conditions, which are collectively common in the UK. Approximately one in three people will develop cancer and one in four will die from it. Many more will be touched by cancer as relatives, friends or carers of cancer patients. Tackling cancer is thus a very high priority in this country.

Cancer also forms part or all of the workload for multiple different healthcare professionals including doctors, nurses, pharmacists, allied health professionals and biomedical scientists. In the community GPs and community nurses have important roles throughout the care pathway. In hospitals a wide range of different specialists contribute to cancer care. These include physicians, surgeons, gynaecologists, pathologists, radiologists and haematologists as well as oncologists and palliative care specialists.

Considerable progress has been made on cancer over the past few years. Death rates are falling year on year and survival rates for several common cancers are improving. In 1970 the five year survival rate for women with breast cancer was around 50%. A patient diagnosed today has around an 80% chance of surviving five years. Over the same period survival rates for bowel cancer have improved from around 25% to around 58%.

In addition to this, large scale surveys have shown that patients' own report on their experience of care has improved. I believe this reflects the spread of multi-disciplinary team working. Within these teams clinical nurse specialists have a critical role in the provision of information, support and continuity of care.

This is an exciting time for everyone who is interested in cancer. New approaches to diagnosis and staging, such as PET-CT scanning have become available. Surgical techniques are being improved and modern radiotherapy equipment can target treatment ever more precisely. Novel targeted systemic therapies are now showing their value, with many more in the pipeline. However, we also need to respond to new challenges, including the increase in incidence of cancer with an ageing population and the rising expectations of patients.

One of the key challenges in tackling cancer is to ensure that all the relevant staff groups have the necessary knowledge and skills. This core text on oncology will help to fill the knowledge gap. It has been written by a multidisciplinary team of experts in the field of cancer and will, I believe, appeal to many different healthcare professionals involved in cancer care. It is both comprehensive and easy to read. The combination of standard text with bullet points, complemented by case histories and 'test yourself' boxes should appeal to people with different learning styles.

I highly recommend this textbook.

Professor Mike Richards CBE
National Cancer Director

Contents

Cancer epidemiology and prevention

'The best sentence in the English language is not "I love you" but "It's benign"'.
Woody Allen 1935– *Deconstructing Harry* (1998 Film)

Introduction

Cancer is a major cause of morbidity and mortality across the world.

Currently in the UK one person in three will be diagnosed with cancer during their lifetime and one in four die of cancer.

In the UK approximately one-quarter of a million people are diagnosed with cancer and 120,000 die each year.

As 60% of all cancers are diagnosed in those aged over 65 years, our rapidly increasing older population suggests that cancer will become an even more common problem in the coming decades.

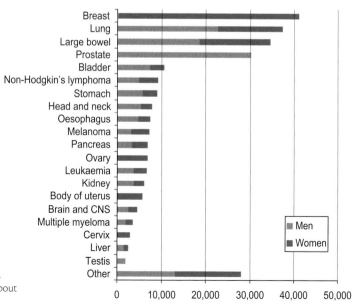

Fig. 1.1 The 20 most commonly diagnosed cancers in the UK. Cancer Research UK, 2006, February, http://www.cancerresearchuk.org/about cancer/statistics/statsmisc/pdfs/ cancerstats_incidence_apr05.pdf.

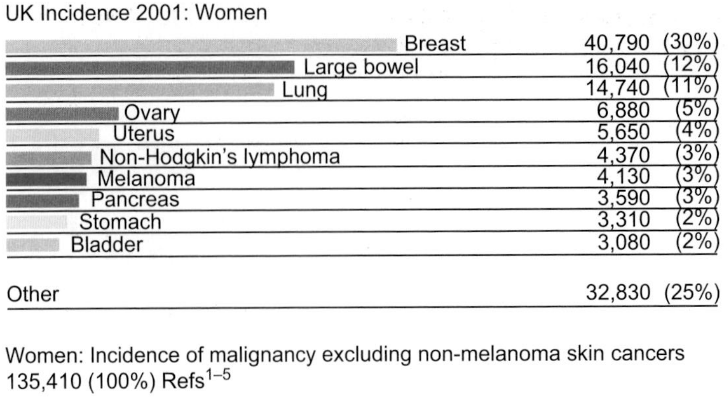

UK Incidence 2001: Women

Breast	40,790 (30%)
Large bowel	16,040 (12%)
Lung	14,740 (11%)
Ovary	6,880 (5%)
Uterus	5,650 (4%)
Non-Hodgkin's lymphoma	4,370 (3%)
Melanoma	4,130 (3%)
Pancreas	3,590 (3%)
Stomach	3,310 (2%)
Bladder	3,080 (2%)
Other	32,830 (25%)

Fig. 1.2 In UK women the most common cancers are those of breast, lung, colon, and skin. Based on data from Cancer Research UK, 2006.

Women: Incidence of malignancy excluding non-melanoma skin cancers 135,410 (100%) Refs[1-5]

UK Incidence 2001: Men

Prostate	30,140 (22%)
Lung	22,700 (17%)
Large bowel	18,500 (14%)
Bladder	7,580 (6%)
Stomach	5,790 (4%)
Head and neck	5,390 (4%)
Non-Hodgkin's lymphoma	4,910 (4%)
Oesophagus	4,680 (3%)
Kidney	3,840 (3%)
Leukaemla	3,830 (3%)
Other	28,010 (20%)

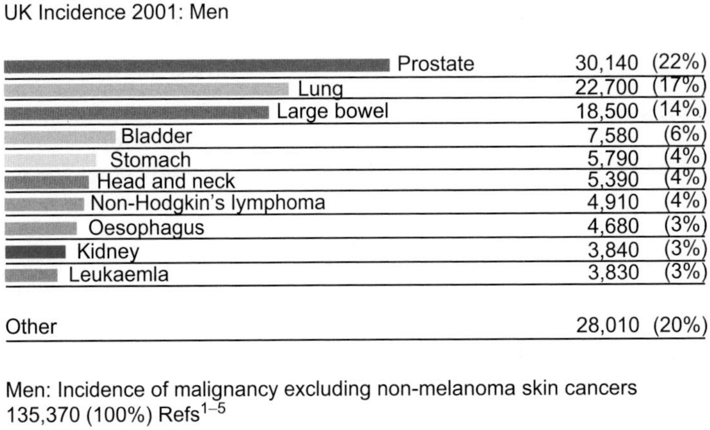

Fig. 1.3 In UK men the commonest cancers are those of the prostate, lung, gastrointestinal tract, and skin. Based on data from Cancer Research UK, 2006.

Men: Incidence of malignancy excluding non-melanoma skin cancers 135,370 (100%) Refs[1-5]

Stop and Think

Will I get cancer?
An individual's risk of developing cancer depends on many factors such as genetic inheritance, smoking behaviour, and diet. However, it is now clear that the cause of cancer is not due to one single event, but is multifactorial.

Incidence

There are huge variations in cancer incidences across the globe, reflecting the impact of environmental and genetic factors on the causes of cancer.[6]

Survival rates

♦ The survival rates for all cancers have risen steadily over the last 20 years

♦ The 5-year relative survival rates for all cancers rose from 18% to 29% for men and from 33% to 43% for women between 1970 and 1990

♦ Overall survival is generally higher for women than men

♦ In women the leading causes of death due to cancer are lung, breast, and colorectal

♦ In men the leading causes of death due to cancer are lung, prostate, and colorectal

♦ Amongst adults, relative survival is lower for elderly patients than for younger patients for almost all cancers

TABLE 1.1 Estimates of the percentage of the population who will develop cancer over a lifetime and the lifetime risk

Site	%	Risk
Men		
Lung	9.1	1 in 11
Skin (non-melanoma)	5.7	1 in 18
Prostate	4.4	1 in 23
Bladder	2.8	1 in 35
Colon	2.6	1 in 38
Stomach	2.4	1 in 42
Rectum	2.0	1 in 50
Non-Hodgkin's lymphoma	1.1	1 in 93
Pancreas	1.1	1 in 95
Oesophagus	1.0	1 in 96
Women		
Breast	11	1 in 9
Skin (non-melanoma)	5.0	1 in 20
Lung	3.8	1 in 26
Colon	3.1	1 in 33
Ovary	1.8	1 in 55
Rectum	1.5	1 in 67
Cervix	1.4	1 in 72
Stomach	1.4	1 in 72
Uterus	1.3	1 in 75
Bladder	1.1	1 in 93

Key Fact

There are more than 200 different types of cancer, but four of them – breast, lung, large bowel (colorectal), and prostate – account for over half of all new cases.

Test Yourself

List the reasons why survival rates for cancers may have improved.

- Financial or material deprivation in adults is linked to worse cancer survival rates. This is not replicated in children

TABLE 1.2 Global incidence of cancer by type

Cancer type	Ratio high/low rate	High incidence	Low incidence
Oesophagus	200:1	Kazakhstan	The Netherlands
Skin	200:1	Australia	India
Liver	100:1	Mozambique	UK
Nasopharynx	100:1	China	Uganda
Lung	40:1	UK	Nigeria
Stomach	30:1	Japan	UK
Cervix	20:1	Hawaii	Israel
Rectum	20:1	Denmark	Nigeria

Key Facts

Cancers are grouped into three survival bands: 50% and over, 10–49% and less than 10%. Of the 20 cancers studied, seven cancers in women (49% of all cancers diagnosed in women) fell into the highest survival category, compared with five cancers for men (30% of all cancers diagnosed in men). For most types of cancer women have a small survival advantage over men.

TABLE 1.3 Global variation in cancer mortality

Country	Number of new cases per year	Number of deaths per year	Cancer deaths: % of new cases
European Union	1,550,806	925,146	60%
Italy	250,508	147,455	59%
Sweden	39,681	20,707	52%
United Kingdom	241,875	155,807	65%

(Adapted from WHO database 2001)

Stop and Think

Why is there such a wide variety in survival rates in patients who have the same cancer but are treated in different countries?

Survival statistics

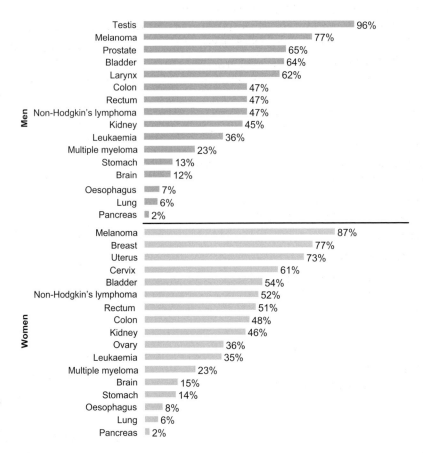

Fig. 1.4 Five-year age standardized relative survival (%), adults diagnosed 1996–1999, England and Wales by sex and site (http://www.cancerresearchuk.org).

International comparisons

Outcomes for patients with cancer have a wide variation when rates between different countries have been compared.

It is important that the most rigorous statistical analysis of the data collected is applied to ensure that confounding factors do not skew the figures, and to make meaningful comparison of scientific papers possible.

In the UK the following conclusions from such comparisons have been drawn:

- Surgeons treating large numbers of patients tend to produce better results than those treating fewer patients
- Children with cancer do better when treated in specialist centres
- Patients with particular cancers (breast, ovary, oesophagus, pancreas, stomach, testis, and lung carcinoma) appear to survive longer when treated at specialist centres

- Patients who are in clinical trials may do better than patients not in trials

These observations motivated the production of the Calman–Hine report into the provision of cancer treatment in the UK. This report's recommendations have had a profound effect on the delivery of cancer care throughout the UK, with the creation of regional cancer centres and local cancer units.

Regional cancer centres serve a population of at least one million, have radiotherapy services and treat patients with both common and more complex and rarer cancers. They provide:

- Specialist surgical services for all cancer types
- Specialist oncologist services for all cancer types
- Specialist palliative care services
- Intensive and routine chemotherapy
- Sophisticated diagnostic imaging: magnetic resonance imaging (MRI), position emission tomography (PET); spiral computerized tomography (CT), etc.

- Specialist clinical nurse skills in intravenous chemotherapy, palliative care, rehabilitation, psychological support, stoma care, and lymphoedema management
- Multidisciplinary working: physiotherapy, dietetics, speech therapy, occupational therapy, and social services

Cancer units at district/area hospital level look after patients with common cancers not requiring radiotherapy. They provide:

- Surgical subspecialization for the more common cancers requiring surgery
- Medical subspecialization for the more common cancers and delivery of chemotherapy
- Nurse specialists
- Specialist palliative care
- Multidisciplinary working: physiotherapy, dietetics, speech therapy, occupational therapy, and social services

Test Yourself

What are the advantages and disadvantages of having cancer care centralized?

Cancer prevention

Cancer prevention can be divided into two areas.

Primary prevention aims to modify factors that promote or protect against carcinogenesis:

- Smoking cessation
- Dietary modification
- Reducing sun exposure

Secondary prevention aims to detect pre-malignant or early malignant disease:

- Population screening (e.g. breast screening)
- Genetic susceptibility testing
- Regular surveillance of high-risk groups

Stop and Think

When health care systems across the world are willing to spend billions of pounds on the development of chemotherapy agents why is it that relatively little is spent on cancer prevention?

Primary prevention

Epidemiological studies have demonstrated that migrants tend to display cancer rates specific to their new adopted country rather than those of their place of origin. Such trends suggest clearly that factors other than genetic predisposition are implicated and emphasize the potential for cancer prevention by reducing exposure to carcinogens or promoting exposure to protective agents.

Smoking

From the cancer perspective smoking causes 30% of all cancer deaths.

TABLE 1.4 Cancer mortality due to behavioural/environmental factors

Factor	% of cancer deaths
Smoking	30
Diet (incuding obesity)	30
Infectious agents	5
Alcohol	3
Sedentary lifestyle	3
Ultraviolet and ionizing radiation	2
Air pollution	2

Smoking-related cancers include:

- Lung cancer
- Oropharyngeal cancer
- Stomach cancer
- Pancreatic cancer
- Renal cancer
- Bladder cancer
- Liver cancer
- Leukaemia

Key Facts

- Smokers who smoke 1–14 cigarettes per day have eight times the risk of dying from lung cancer compared with a non-smoker
- With > 25 cigarettes per day the risk is 25-fold
- The risk of lung cancer falls by 50% 10 years after and by 90% 15 years after stopping smoking

Diet
Carcinogens

The relationship between certain food types and carcinogenesis is difficult to prove. The majority of potential cancer-causing agents are a natural part of foodstuffs, while others are produced by cooking or microbial contamination.

Examples include:

- Aflatoxins – produced by *Aspergillus* moulds, found on the surface of crops such as groundnuts or maize, have been implicated in the development of hepatocellular cancer
- N-nitroso compounds – these chemicals are found in salted, smoked or pickled meat and have a positive correlation with the development of oesophageal, nasopharyngeal, bladder, and hepatocellular cancer

Dietary fat

Animals receiving diets that are high in saturated fats have an increased incidence of cancer, though it is unclear if it is the high calorific value of fat that makes it a risk factor in cancer.

Obesity and a sedentary life-style are risk factors for:

- Breast cancer
- Colorectal cancer
- Renal cancer
- Endometrial cancer

Fruit and vegetables

The protective effect of fruit and vegetables has been consistently demonstrated though it has been difficult to identify which components of these foods are active in preventing cancer. The cruciferous vegetables (broccoli, cauliflower, and Brussels sprouts) are claimed to be particularly protective.

Alcohol

The mechanism of carcinogenesis is unclear and the close association with smoking complicates population studies.

Alcohol-associated cancers include:

- Oral cavity
- Pharynx
- Oesophagus
- Liver
- Breast

Key Facts

Asbestos

- Asbestos has been used for its heat-resistant properties in the construction and shipbuilding industries
- Both chrysotile (white asbestos) and particularly crocidolite (blue asbestos) are carcinogenic, leading to the development of mesothelioma, typically up to 40 years post-exposure
- Asbestos alone can cause lung cancer but also has a synergistic effect with smoking (fivefold risk)
- The incidence of asbestos-related cancers will rise in coming years because of increasing exposure pre-1980

Occupational carcinogens

In 1775 Sir Percival Pott identified chimney soot as the cause of squamous carcinoma of the scrotum in chimney sweeps. Since then numerous other workplace carcinogens have been identified, the most infamous example being asbestos.

Ultraviolet light

Skin cancer is the most common malignancy seen in Western countries but accounts for just 2% of cancer deaths.

Whether the rising incidence is the result of the fashion for sun-tans or a decrease in the ozone layer with increased ultraviolet B levels is unclear. Excess exposure to sunlight in childhood is especially harmful.

Mechanism

- Squamous cell and basal cell skin carcinomas are associated with cumulative exposure to ultraviolet light
- Malignant melanoma is associated with episodes of acute ultraviolet damage
- The shorter wavelengths (ultraviolet B and C) are most damaging to DNA but even ultraviolet A (often used in sun-beds) causes DNA damage

Cancer Research UK recommendations regarding sun exposure are:

- Avoid the midday sun
- Seek natural shade when in sunlight, e.g. trees
- Wear cover-up clothing, including T-shirts and hats

TABLE 1.5	Examples of virus-associated cancers
Virus	**Cancer**
Hepatitis B, C	Hepatocellular cancer
HIV	Kaposi's sarcoma, lymphoma
Epstein–Barr virus	Nasopharyngeal cancer, Burkitt's lymphoma
Human papillomavirus	Cervical cancer

TABLE 1.6	Diagnosis by screening tests		
Test result	**Disease**	**No disease**
Positive	a	b
Negative	c	d

Sensitivity % = a/(a + c) × 100
Specificity (%) = d/(b – d) × 100
Positive predictive value % – a/(a + b) × 100

- Use a broad-spectrum sunscreen of sun protection factor 15 or higher. Sun protection factor is seen as a guide to how much longer it is possible to stay in the sun before becoming burned

- Re-apply sunscreen frequently

- Especially protect children from sun exposure

Virus-related cancers

World-wide over 850,000 cases of cancer per year are attributable to viral infection (Table 1.5).

Prevention possibilities include:

- Vaccination programmes against hepatitis B

- Education programmes aimed at reducing high-risk sexual activity

Congenital or genetic abnormalities

Certain congenital or genetic abnormalities are associated with a high risk of cancer development. Sometimes prophylactic surgery can be offered.

Examples of surgical cancer prevention include:

- Orchidopexy to prevent testicular cancer in cryptorchidism

- Colectomy to avoid cancer in patients with hereditary colorectal cancer or ulcerative colitis but especially Familial adenomatous polyposis coli (FAP) where there is a 100% risk that polyps eventually turn malignant

- Bilateral mastectomy in patients with familial breast cancer

Stop and Think

Has reading about the ways in which it is possible to decrease your risk of getting cancer made you change any of your habits? If not, why not? Would it influence your future patients?

- Laparoscopic oophorectomy in women with familial ovarian cancer

Secondary prevention

The validity of a screening test can be defined as its ability to correctly identify individuals who have a disease and those who do not. It consists of three components.

Sensitivity

This is the test's ability to correctly identify those individuals with disease. If the test is not sufficiently sensitive, then many individuals who have cancer will be wrongly reassured by **a false-negative result**.

Specificity

This is the test's ability to correctly identify those individuals who do not have disease.

The screening test must be sufficiently specific to prevent undue anxiety in a large number of individuals who are given **a false-positive result** but do not have cancer.

Positive predictive value

This is a measure of the reliability of a positive test result indicating true disease.

Screening tests with a high positive predictive value lead to fewer unnecessary follow-up investigations.

Screening for breast cancer

- Mammography is the only breast cancer screening method that has been shown to reduce mortality

- It is highly specific (90%) and sensitive (90%) in detecting breast cancer in post-menopausal women

- The UK programme is believed to prevent 1,250 deaths a year

- A reduction in mortality of 25% has been shown in women over the age of 50

- In the UK, routine screening 3-yearly is currently offered to women aged 50–64. There are plans to extend the age of screening up to 69 from 2006.

Key Facts

Mammography and hormone replacement therapy (HRT)
There has recently been a survey of all the studies into the relationship between the use of HRT and the effectiveness of mammography, which concluded that it is more difficult to interpret the mammograms of women using HRT.

More women who are on HRT are likely to get either false-negative (missing a cancer which is there) or false-positive (suspecting a cancer which turns out not to be there) results for their mammograms compared to women who do not take HRT.

Women older than the upper age limit can have mammograms performed every 3 years on request

- A positive result is followed by a fine-needle aspiration or core biopsy, if need be under radiological guidance

- In women under the age of 50 consistent benefit from screening has not been demonstrated

Problems include:

- Compliance may be poor, as 80% of women find the procedure uncomfortable (UK compliance is 70%)

- False-positive results occur in 1% of cases causing unnecessary anxiety (10% of women screened are recalled after the initial mammogram for further investigations)

- Breast tumours can occur in the time interval between scans (16 per 10,000 women screened)

Young women with a family history of disease tend to be first screened 10 years before their youngest affected relative was diagnosed. This can be difficult because mammograms are insensitive in younger women with more dense breast tissue. MRI is an alternative screening tool in this situation.

Screening for cervical cancer

Cancer of the uterine cervix is the second most common cancer in middle-aged women (after breast cancer) and the detection and treatment of its precancerous

Key Fact

Women with familial autosomal dominant breast cancer are likely to have earlier age of onset and bilateral disease.

state can modify its outcome. Cervical screening has been shown, retrospectively, to be successful in reducing cancer deaths in several countries.

- Around 1,500 UK women died in the year 2000 from invasive cervical cancer. This has decreased from over 2000 per year in 1971

- Screening is carried out 5-yearly for women from the ages of 20 to 64

- 85% of women in the target group comply with screening due to excellent GP programmes

- Unfortunately, women in lower socioeconomic groups, who are at the highest risk of developing cancer, often do not comply with screening

Abnormal smear tests are reported as a grade of cellular abnormality (dyskaryosis). Follow-up depends on the severity of the abnormality:

- **Borderline or mild dyskaryosis**: repeat smear 6 months later and if still abnormal colposcopy is performed. A minimum of two consecutive negative smears 6 months apart are needed after a borderline or mildly dyskaryotic result before standard screening can be resumed

- **Moderate and severe dyskaryosis**: refer for colposcopy immediately

Colposcopy allows direct identification and biopsy of carcinoma *in situ* (CIS):

- If grade I CIS is present, this can be kept under surveillance, as a proportion of these changes will revert to normal

- If grade II or grade III CIS is identified, immediate local treatment is required

The human papillomavirus (HPV) is a cofactor in cervical cancer development.

- A strong association with HPV types 16 and 18 has been noted

- A possible primary preventative measure for the future may be HPV vaccination

- This, however, will not prevent all cervical cancers, as some do not appear to be associated with viral infection

Screening for colorectal cancer

There is good evidence from clinical trials that faecal occult blood testing every 2 years followed by colonoscopy or flexible sigmoidoscopy in those who are positive will allow the early detection of colorectal cancer.

Future Possibilities

In the future, virtual colonoscopy may be the method of choice to follow-up positive faecal occult bloods. In this method, a CT scan of the abdomen is carried out and a computer reconstructs images of the bowel wall. The procedure takes less than 1 minute but interpretation may take longer.

Key Fact

Prostatic cancer screening
Until such times as we have a better understanding of prostatic cancer's natural history and its optimum treatment in the early stages, screening should only be undertaken within the context of a clinical trial.

With a compliance rate of 60%, screening of 50–69-year-olds would be expected to prevent 1,200 deaths per year in the UK.

Before faecal occult blood analysis can be carried out the patient must be taking a special diet. This, and a false-positive result rate of 10%, may reduce patient compliance.

Faecal occult blood testing has a positive predictive value of 50%. This means for every 10 people who test positive, five will have significant findings, including but not exclusively cancer, on further investigation.

At present two methods are being considered:

♦ **Flexible sigmoidoscopy** has a sensitivity of 80%

♦ **Full colonoscopy**, also with a sensitivity of 80%, although some experts have reported tumour detection rates of 90–100%

In summary, colorectal screening has proven benefit in cancer prevention in several trials. There are financial and manpower issues, as well as concerns about patient compliance, to be resolved prior to its introduction. However, in 2005 the UK Government gave approval *in principle* to just such a screening programme, beginning in England 2006/7.

Prostatic cancer screening

In the UK, 10,000 men each year die from prostatic cancer and this figure is rising annually.

Efforts to develop a secondary prevention of cancer screening test for middle-aged men have been attempted but results have been disappointing.

Screening modalities used to date include the following:

♦ **Digital rectal examination** – this was traditionally used prior to 1990. Unfortunately, despite annual tests, only 20% of those men having an abnormal rectal examination had localized disease which could be cured by early treatment. Of men with metastatic disease, 25% had a normal prostatic examination. This method is therefore of low sensitivity and low specificity and is not used as a screening tool.

♦ **Transrectal ultrasound** – when this was evaluated as a screening test it proved to be insensitive and non-specific. It is, however, used in the evaluation of patients with proven prostatic cancer

♦ **Prostatic-specific antigen** – an elevated prostate-specific antigen (PSA) of over 4 ng/ml predicts prostatic cancer with a sensitivity of 71% and a specificity of 91%. This makes PSA a potential screening modality

Currently PSA screening is *not* recommended by the UK Department of Health because:

♦ A beneficial outcome from early detection of the disease has not been proven

♦ The frequency of prostatic cancers found at autopsy steadily increases for each decade over 50 years and most of these tumours are clinically silent

♦ Detecting early prostatic cancers may cause unnecessary anxiety, along with the significant morbidity and mortality associated with surgery or radiotherapy, of unknown benefit

Other tumours undergoing evaluation for potential screening, but not as yet in a national programme, include ovarian carcinoma (ultrasound – UK) and high risk groups for lung cancer (spiral CT – USA).

Surveillance

Surveillance is secondary cancer prevention offered to individuals known to be at high risk of malignancy. It must be distinguished from screening that is applied to a population at large.

Examples:

♦ Regular colonoscopy in patients with ulcerative colitis or familial colorectal cancer

♦ Patients with a strong family history of breast cancer are recommended to have regular surveillance mammography. This should start 10 years before the age of onset of cancer in the youngest affected family member. In young women MRI is more sensitive than mammography

TABLE 1.7 Genetic susceptibility tests in use

Hereditary cancer syndrome	Gene mutations identifiable
Breast and ovarian cancer	BRCA1, BRCA2?, BRCA3?, BRCA4
Hereditary non-polyposis coli	MSH2, MLH2, PMS2, PMS1, MSH6
Familial adenomatous polyposis coli	APC
Multiple endocrine neoplasia type 1	MEN1
Multiple endocrine neoplasia type 2	RET
von Hippel–Lindau disease	VHL
Retinoblastoma	RBI
Li–Fraumeni syndrome.	P53
Melanoma	P16, CDK4

Genetic susceptibility testing

In families with hereditary cancer syndromes, an increasing number of associated genetic abnormalities are being recognized. Testing for these genetic mutations allows the physician to identify individuals in a family at high risk of developing cancer.

Chapter summary

- With an increasing elderly population the number of patients with cancer is likely to increase
- Five cancers – lung, colorectal, breast, skin and prostate – account for more than 50% of cancer diagnoses in the UK
- Survival rates for patients with the same cancer differ widely from country to country
- Primary cancer prevention attempts to influence factors that promote or protect against carcinogenesis
- Secondary cancer prevention aims to detect pre-malignant or early malignant disease
- Surveillance is secondary cancer prevention applied to particular individuals who are known to be at high risk of malignancy
- Smoking is responsible for 30% of cancer deaths, with clear and direct evidence of causation
- Diet may be responsible for up to 30% of cancer deaths but the evidence of clear causation is much less clear than for smoking

Key Facts

BRCA1 and BRCA2 testing

- A woman with a BRCA1 or BRCA2 mutation faces about a 60–85% lifetime risk of breast cancer and a 20–60% risk of ovarian cancer
- Genetic testing in families with a strong family history of breast or ovarian cancer may allow prevention of some of these malignancies
- The current difficulty is that there are no recognized primary interventions for BRCA1 or BRCA2 mutations

Possible measures include:

- **Prophylactic surgery** – bilateral mastectomies and laparoscopic oophorectomies have been suggested to reduce the risk of breast and ovarian cancer but have not been proven in large randomized trials
  - Surgery reduces (by 95%) but does not eliminate the risk of cancer and may be associated with considerable psychological morbidity.
- **Chemoprevention** – tamoxifen* for prevention of breast cancer or low-dose oestrogen for reducing risk of ovarian cancer are under investigation but, again, these are controversial

*The British and European view is that tamoxifen should not be used in this circumstance outwith a controlled trial whereas in the USA tamoxifen is more widely used for prophylaxis despite the known side effects (stroke, pulmonary emboli, endometrial polyps and malignancy).

- At present, BRCA1 and BRCA2 testing in high-risk individuals may be of value in guiding secondary rather than primary prevention in the form of regular mammography, transvaginal ultrasound and CA-125 levels
- Legal issues regarding the disclosure of BRCA1 or BRCA2 status to financial or insurance companies will become important
- As there are possible long-term implications for the individual and her relatives, counselling and informed consent are essential before genetic testing

'Susceptibility testing' differs from screening in that:

- It is only applied to a small, high-risk group rather than the population at large
- It is only performed once
- It is usually expensive
- The potential ramifications require skilled counselling before testing on the implications of taking a 'gene test'

When a positive result is obtained, the physician may then offer primary cancer prevention (such as chemoprevention or surgery), or may recommend secondary prevention in the form of regular surveillance (such as colonoscopy in hereditary colorectal tumours or mammography in *BRCA* mutations). *BRCA1* and *BRCA2* testing is being used increasingly within the UK.

References

1. Office for National Statistics. *Cancer statistics registrations: Registrations of cancer diagnosed in 2000, England.* (1. Series MB1 no.31.): National Statistics, 2003. London
2. ISD Online. *Cancer Incidence and Mortality.* NHS Scotland.
3. Welsh Cancer Intelligence and Surveillance Unit, 2003.
4. Northern Ireland Cancer Registry 2004, Cancer Incidence and Mortality.
5. http://www.cancerresearchuk.org
6. Souhami RL, Tobias JD. *Cancer and its management,* 5th edition Oxford: Blackwell Science, 2005.

Pathogenesis of cancer

Cancer development

Cancers may develop in any body tissue.

Cancerous cells can be distinguished from cells in normal tissues in a number of ways.

They may exhibit:

- Cell division that has escaped the control of normal homeostasis
- Abnormalities of cell differentiation – in general terms, cancer cells tend to be less well differentiated than their non-malignant counterparts
- Resistance to programmed cell death or apoptosis
- The potential to invade local tissues and metastasize

The cause of cancer is multifactorial and includes life-style, environmental exposures, and inherited genetic susceptibility. It is thought that as many as 80–90% of all cancers may be the result of such environmental or life-style factors. Changes to the individual's genome are increasingly thought to be the *final common pathway* in the development of cancer, whatever the initial trigger. These genetic influences are often classified as initiators or promoters.

The Human Genome Project (completed in 2003) has shown the DNA sequence for 30,000 genes. However, linking genes to the risks of disease with certainty is far from the straightforward process that is sometimes portrayed in the popular media, as there are many other complex environmental factors involved.

Key Facts

Genetic influences

- The **initiation** step is usually rapid, irreversible and the result of DNA damage (i.e. mutations, caused by chemical carcinogens, radiation, or viruses)

- **Promotion** describes the step in which there is proliferation and clonal expansion of initiated cells. In contrast to initiators, promoters do not affect the DNA directly and their effects are reversible. The initiator must be applied before the promoter; there may be a long delay before application of the promoter. The promoter must be applied repeatedly and at regular intervals

---

The development of cancer is associated with the accumulation of defects or 'mutations' in a number of critical genes within the cell. Many cancers, for example, are associated with mutations leading to 'overactivity' of growth-promoting genes, known commonly as oncogenes. Conversely, cancers may also be associated with mutations leading to 'underactivity' of genes which act to suppress growth.

Chemical cancer initiation

A variety of natural and synthetic compounds that initiate carcinogenesis have been identified. They fall into two groups:

- **Direct** – compounds which are themselves carcinogenic

- **Indirect** – compounds or pro-carcinogens which are metabolically converted *in vivo* to the actual carcinogen

Chemicals that are capable of transforming a cell are highly reactive electrophiles, i.e. they have electron-deficient atoms that can react with nucleophilic (electron-rich) sites within the cell. Although the primary target within the cell for these electrophilic reactions is DNA, other electron-rich sites such as RNA and proteins will also be attacked. This will sometimes be lethal to the cell, but if not the DNA damage will be transmitted to daughter cells and perpetuated in subsequent generations of cells. In an effort to prevent this, cellular DNA repair mechanisms attempt to reconstitute the DNA before cell division.

Chemical cancer promotion

The process of promotion, in contrast to initiation, is gradual, partially reversible, and requires prolonged exposure to the promoting agent. Promoters do not need to be metabolized to the active compound; they have no tendency to react as electrophiles and they rarely induce tumours themselves. When a cell that has undergone initiation is exposed to a promoter, that cell is stimulated to divide and the number of genetically damaged cells increases. With continued cell division there is selection for those cells that have an increased growth rate and enhanced invasive properties as a

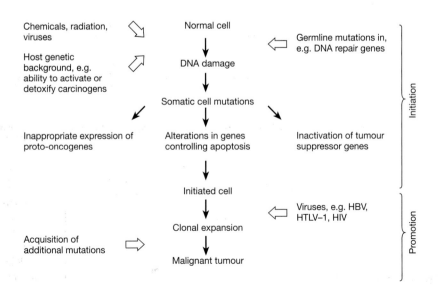

Fig. 2.1 General scheme for carcinogenesis in which promoters cause clonal expansion of the initiated cell.

result of genetic mutation. Promotion can, therefore, be regarded as stimulating the proliferation of pre-neoplastic cells, malignant conversion, and tumour progression. At each step of this multistep process, additional mutations are acquired by the initiated cell, resulting in the formation of a malignant tumour. Promoters are non-mutagenic and contribute to tumorigenesis by induction of cell proliferation mechanisms.

Radiation

There are many similarities in the basic mode of action of chemical and radiation-induced carcinogenesis. As with most chemical carcinogens, radiation is mutagenic and thought to cause malignant transformation by DNA damage. There are usually many years between exposure to the initiating dose of radiation and the appearance of malignancy. This would suggest that exposure to promoting agents is involved in proliferation of radiation-damaged cells and ultimate tumour development.

Ultraviolet radiation

Ultraviolet (UV) radiation of the appropriate wavelength can be absorbed by DNA bases and generate changes in them. The UV portion of the solar spectrum can be divided into three wavelength ranges: UVA (320–400 nm), UVB (280–320 nm) and UVC (200–280 nm). UVB is thought to be responsible for the induction of cutaneous cancers through DNA damage. This type of DNA damage is normally repaired by the nucleotide excision repair pathway. The five steps in this pathway are:

- Recognition of the DNA lesion
- Incision of the DNA strand on both sides of the lesion
- Removal of the damaged strand
- Synthesis of a nucleotide patch
- Ligation of the patch to adjacent nucleotides

The importance of the excision repair pathway is observed in patients with the autosomal recessive disorder xeroderma pigmentosum, who have an inherited inability to repair UV-induced DNA damage. Such patients demonstrate extreme photosensitivity and

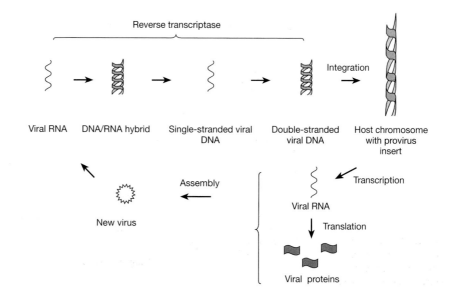

Fig. 2.2 Retroviral life cycle.

have a 2,000-fold increased risk of skin cancer in sun-exposed skin. Xeroderma pigmentosum is genetically heterogeneous with at least seven different variants, each of which is caused by a mutation in one of several genes involved in the excision repair pathway.

Viral factors

A number of DNA and RNA viruses have now been implicated in human tumours. They cause transformation by integrating their genome into the host cell DNA. Usually the virus is responsible for the production of a *transforming protein*, coded by an oncogene, which maintains the transformed state within the cell.

* DNA tumour viruses – the oncogene is an integral part of the viral genome
* RNA tumour viruses – may be of viral origin or may be a host gene that is inappropriately expressed following viral infection

Key Facts

HIV

The human immunodeficiency virus (HIV) is a retrovirus that induces acquired immunodeficiency syndrome (AIDS) which then leads to a variety of different tumours. These are of two main types:

* Those which are related to immunosuppression, e.g. following Epstein–Barr virus infection in which the virus is released from its normal immune control
* Those that probably develop as a result of growth factors released from HIV-infected cells, e.g. Kaposi's sarcoma in which plaques or nodules appear on skin and mucosa; multiple lesions are regarded as being independent in origin rather than as a result of metastasis

Chapter summary

* The causes of cancer are multifactorial
* Up to 90% of cancers may be caused by environmental or life-style factors
* Initiation (with damage to DNA) followed by promotion (with proliferation of initiated cells) are thought to represent the pathway for the development of many cancers
* Cancers may be linked to mutations leading to overactivity of growth-promoting genes or under-activity of genes which suppress growth
* Chemical carcinogens are usually electron-deficient and react with nucleophilic electron-rich DNA and RNA
* Radiation is mutagenic but it usually takes many years of exposure to promoting agents before proliferation of radiation-damaged cells leads to tumour development
* Viruses are implicated in tumour formation by integrating their own genome into the host DNA

CHAPTER 3

Diagnosis, staging, treatment intent, and planning

Early clinical detection

Early detection of cancer is crucial in improving the patient's chances of successful treatment. Early clinical detection means diagnosing the cancer when it is localized and has not developed regional or distant spread to lymph nodes or other tissues.

Clinical symptoms and signs of cancer

Cancer normally presents with signs or symptoms as a result of changes in normal physiological function. A cancer can cause signs or symptoms either locally at the original site, or once it has spread elsewhere in the body. The local signs and symptoms will depend on where the cancer started. For example, a patient with lung cancer may present with cough, haemoptysis, or breathlessness. If that patient's cancer has spread elsewhere, they may have distant signs and symptoms such as pain from bone metastases or weight and appetite loss related to liver metastases. These non-specific signs and symptoms are often only recognized as having been heralds of malignancy in retrospect.

> **Stop and Think**
>
> **Difficulties of general practice**
> Less than 3% of patients who present with rectal bleeding to their GP will have cancer.

Cancer detection, diagnosis, and staging

Once cancer is suspected, the diagnosis must be confirmed or excluded, usually by obtaining a histological biopsy. If a positive diagnosis is made the extent of the diagnosis must be determined by further investigations.

Establishing that a cancer is present does not provide enough information to start treatment. The temptation to jump to therapeutic decisions must be resisted until an accurate and comprehensive assessment of the patient and their disease has been made. The more that is known about the tumour and the patient, the greater the likelihood that the most effective treatment can be given.

Key elements in accurate diagnosis and staging

The *histological nature* of the particular tumour is usually determined after fine-needle biopsy, core biopsy, surgical biopsy, or excision of a mass.

The *extent of spread of tumour* requires clinical, radiological, biochemical, and sometimes surgical assessment.

Histological assessment

Expert pathological input is vital in cancer diagnosis and treatment. The pathologist will aim to confirm that a lesion is indeed malignant and also confirm the tissue in which the cancer originated. It is important to know whether the cancer has been fully excised, what the grade is (i.e. whether it appears more or less aggressive),

and any special molecular or biochemical features that may influence treatment.

Radiological imaging

Marked improvements in non-invasive or minimally invasive imaging techniques have greatly reduced the need for surgical staging. However, laparoscopic assessment of intra-abdominal tumours, such as stomach or ovarian cancer, may detect small peritoneal secondaries and thus radically alter treatment strategies.

An increasing number of medical imaging procedures exist to detect cancer. These include:

- Plain or contrast radiography
- Computerized tomography (CT)
- Radioisotope scanning
- Ultrasound (US)
- Magnetic resonance imaging (MRI)
- Arteriography
- Positron emission tomography (PET)

MRI and CT techniques are non-invasive techniques that can produce cross-sectional pictures of the body to show the shape, size, and location of a tumour. They are important in staging patients and in assessing response to treatment. The ability to create three-dimensional images also permits better staging and planning for surgery and radiation therapy. Whilst CT is generally preferred to MRI when evaluating the lungs and abdominal cavity, MRI is superior for imaging the mediastinum, liver, and pelvis. Both can be used to examine the brain, but MRI is more sensitive and can also be used to assess the spinal cord.

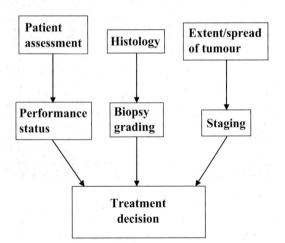

Fig. 3.1 Diagram of process of diagnosis and staging.

> **Key Facts**
>
> **Spiral CT**
> A spiral (or helical) CT scan is a new kind of CT. During spiral CT, the X-ray machine rotates continuously around the body, following a spiral path to make cross-sectional pictures of the body. Benefits of spiral CT include:
>
> - It can be used to make three–dimensional pictures of areas inside the body
> - It may detect small abnormal areas better than conventional CT
> - It is faster, so the test takes less time than conventional CT

Stop and Think

CT scan risks

A CT examination has a radiation dose that may be associated with an increase in the possibility of fatal cancer of approximately 1 chance in 2000. This increase in the possibility of a fatal cancer from radiation can be compared to the natural incidence of fatal cancer in the UK population (about 1 chance in 4). In other words, for any one person the risk of radiation-induced cancer is much smaller than the natural risk of cancer. Nevertheless, this small increase in radiation-associated cancer risk for an individual can become a public health concern if large numbers of the population undergo increased numbers of CT screening procedures of uncertain benefit. http://www.pueblo.gsa.gov/cic_text/health/fullbody-ctscan/risks.htm

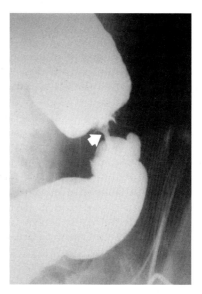

Fig. 3.3 Contrast study
A spot view from a barium enema in a patient with a history of rectal bleeding shows the typical appearance of a cancer involving the descending colon. There is marked concentric narrowing of the bowel lumen with associated shouldering of the edges, giving the typical apple-core appearance of a bowel cancer (arrow).

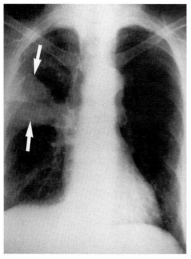

Fig. 3.2 Plain radiograph
Frontal chest radiograph of an elderly patient who presented with haemoptysis. The patient was a heavy smoker. The radiograph shows a large shadow (arrows) extending from the right hilum to the periphery of the lung. The mass was biopsied percutaneously by a radiologist and was shown to represent a primary lung cancer.

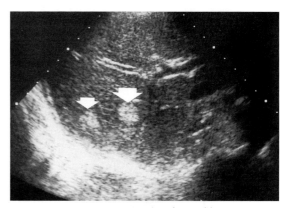

Fig. 3.4 Ultrasound (US)
Seen in a 51-year-old woman with abdominal distension. US shows bilateral adnexal masses, massive free fluid and seeding along the broad ligament. Laparotomy revealed multiple metastases attached to the abdominal wall. Arrows point to adnexal masses.

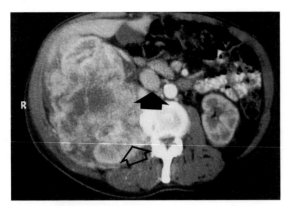

Fig. 3.5 Computerized tomography (CT)
Axial CT scan of a middle-aged man who presented with
haematuria. The scans were performed through the level of the
kidneys following the injection of intravenous contrast. There is a
large mass involving the right kidney. There is marked enhancement
of the mass, indicating hypervascularity. The right psoas muscle is
directly invaded by the tumour (open arrow). The inferior vena cava
is displaced anteriorly by the mass (closed arrow). The mass was
confirmed histologically as renal cell carcinoma. The presence of
local muscle invasion carries a poor prognosis.

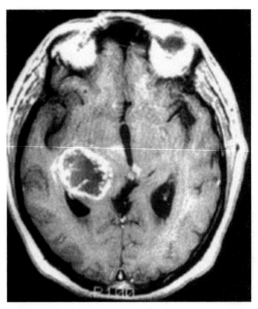

Fig. 3.7 Magnetic resonance imaging (MRI)
Glioblastoma multiforme – MRI scan showing tumour in frontal
lobe http://www.sd-neurosurgeon.com/diseases/glioblastoma.html

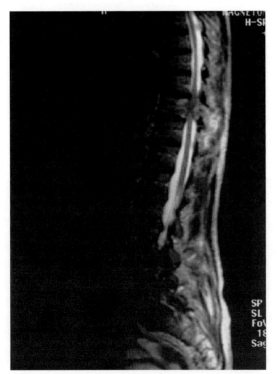

Fig. 3.6 Magnetic resonance imaging (MRI) (normal sagittal view).
The two major advantages of MRI over other imaging modalities are
its lack of ionizing radiation and its ability to view anatomy and
pathology in multiple planes. T1-weighted images best demonstrate
anatomy. T2-weighted images best demonstrate pathological
conditions because most inflammatory and neoplastic processes
appear bright in signal as a result of their increased water content.
Image shows spinal cord lesion.

Future Possibilities

Positron emission tomography (PET)

PET is increasingly used for tumour localization
and follow-up. PET scanning uses positron-emitting
isotopes of oxygen, nitrogen, carbon, fluorine, and
rubidium. Positrons are particles identical to elec-
trons except that they are positively charged. Positrons travel a short distance, giving up kinetic energy
by Compton interactions, and finally colliding with a
free electron, resulting in total annihilation. It is the
photons from the total annihilation of the positron
and electron that are detected by PET scanning. A ring
of detectors is placed around the area to be imaged
which picks up the energy released from the annihilation process. Since each annihilation originates
from a specific point in space, an image is generated
which contains spatial information.

PET does not offer such high resolution as CT or
MRI but provides functional and metabolic information. One of the commonest agents used in PET scanning is 5-FDG (fluorinated deoxyglucose). Because
glucose is so avidly taken up by actively dividing cells
such as cancer cells, 5-FDG tends to collect in cancer
cells, so that tumours are shown as bright spots. PET
may, therefore, help to distinguish benign from
malignant lesions and can be helpful in deciding
whether a residual mass after cancer therapy represents fibrosis or residual tumour.

Goals of cancer staging

Clinical decisions regarding the treatment of a particular patient are based upon the histological diagnosis and anatomical extent or stage of the cancer.

The objectives of cancer staging and histological classification are:

- To allow the clinician to determine the aim of treatment (palliative or curative)
- To aid the clinician in planning the type of treatment
- To give some indication of prognosis for the patient
- To evaluate the efficacy of treatment by repeating investigations following therapy
- To assist in clinical trials

Staging depends on measuring and defining the extent of the disease.

The tumour stage is a reflection of the tumour burden and is determined by three major criteria which are:

- **T** – primary tumour
- **N** – regional lymph node
- **M** – metastases

The TNM classification defines the primary site as T_1-T_4 with increasing size of the primary lesion, advancing nodal disease as N_0-N_3, and the presence or absence of metastases as M_0 or M_1. The T, N, and M parameters are combined to define a clinically relevant stage of disease. The exact criteria for staging depend on the individual primary organ sites.

A typical type of stage grouping is the following:

Stage 1
Clinical examination revealing a tumour confined to the primary organ. This lesion tends to be operable and completely resectable.

Stage 2
Clinical examination shows evidence of local spread into surrounding tissue and first draining lymph nodes. The lesion is also operable and resectable but there is a higher risk of further spread of the disease.

Stage 3
Clinical examination reveals an extensive primary tumour with fixation to deeper structures and local invasion. This lesion may not be operable and may require a combination of treatment modalities.

Stage 4
Evidence of distant metastases beyond the site of origin. The primary site may be surgically inoperable.

Histopathological staging and classification

Histopathological classification is extremely important in defining the tumour type and for making treatment decisions.

Such classification involves defining the histopathological type or grade (or degree of differentiation).

Tumours may be classified histopathologically by type, for example:

- Adenocarcinoma
- Squamous carcinoma
- Small cell carcinoma
- Large cell carcinoma
- Sarcoma
- Lymphoma
- Leukaemia (myeloid and lymphocytic)
- Glioma
- Seminoma
- Teratoma

The degree of differentiation is classified as:

- Well differentiated
- Moderately differentiated
- Poorly differentiated

Tumour grade is classified as:

- Low grade
- Intermediate grade
- High grade

High-grade, poorly differentiated tumours tend to have a poorer outcome than low-grade, well-differentiated tumours.

Future Possibilities

The particular biochemical, molecular, and genetic characteristics of individual tumours are increasingly important in targeting treatment to a specific tumour.

Blood tests

Routine blood tests may be helpful. For example, in a patient with cancer, abnormal liver biochemistry tests may indicate the presence of liver metastases while a raised alkaline phosphatase and serum calcium may reflect bone metastases.

Tumour markers

Biological markers may also be useful as an adjunct to staging and histological classification of tumours. Tumour markers produced by a cancer, such as carcino-embryonic antigen (CEA), human β-chorionic gonado-trophin (βHCG), alpha-fetoprotein (αFP), prostate-specific antigen (PSA), and CA-125 may contribute to the histo-pathological classification of tumours. Markers such as epithelial membrane antigen and common leucocyte antigen help differentiate between epithelial and lymphoid malignancies. Tumour markers such as CA-125, βHCG, and αFP circulating in the blood may also be useful in monitoring response to treatment.

Principles of cancer treatment

The major principle governing the initial approach to treatment for a cancer patient is to define the goals of clinical management. For those patients with curable disease, the goal is to cure the patient using proven single or combined modality treatments. However, if the cancer is not curable, the goals of treatment are to improve the quality of the patient's life and prolong life (with good quality).

Treatment principles are based upon:

- The preferences of the patient

- The biological behaviour of the cancer

- The mortality and morbidity of the therapeutic procedure

- The efficacy of the therapeutic procedure under consideration

- The performance status (general level of fitness) of the patient

In the treatment of cancer it is important to realize that standard treatments for cancer patients are based upon large clinical studies that have shown improved disease-free and overall survival. The most commonly chosen parameters to measure survival and benefit of treatment are 5-year disease-free and overall survival rates.

- Patients with localized cancers can often be cured

- Patients presenting with positive lymph nodes tend to have poorer prognosis but can be cured

- Patients with distant metastases are rarely cured but in some cases may survive for 5 years with multimodality treatments. Exceptions to this graver prognosis include childhood cancers, haematological malignancies, and germ cell tumours

TABLE 3.1 Eastern Co-operative Oncology Group (ECOG) Performance Status Scale

Fully active; able to carry on all activities without restriction	0
Restricted in physically strenuous activity but ambulatory and able to carry out work of a light or sedentary nature	1
Ambulatory and capable of all self-care; confined to bed or chair 50% of waking hours	2
Capable of only limited self-care; confined to bed or chair 50% or more of waking hours	3
Completely disabled; cannot carry on any self-care; totally confined to bed or chair	4

Key Fact

Performance Status Scale
Patients who have a performance status score greater than two on the ECOG scale usually do not tolerate intensive oncological treatments.

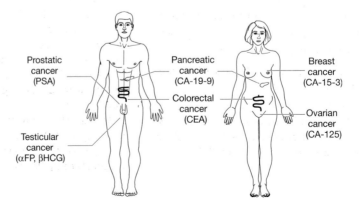

Fig. 3.8 Tumour markers used in the diagnosis and evaluation of cancer (PSA, prostate-specific antigen; CEA, carcinoembryonic antigen; αFP, alpha-fetoprotein; βHCG, β-chorionic gonadotrophin).

Prostatic cancer (PSA)

Testicular cancer (αFP, βHCG)

Pancreatic cancer (CA-19-9)

Colorectal cancer (CEA)

Breast cancer (CA-15-3)

Ovarian cancer (CA-125)

Stop and Think

Communicating difficult information

Before commencing any treatment it is important that the patient, their relatives, and carers are aware of the goals and limitations of treatment.

It is not unusual, after what the consultant feels to have been a very full and frank discussion outlining these goals, for a patient to ask a much more junior member of the team to clarify what has been said. This may be because they do not wish to admit not understanding what was being discussed. Alternatively, they may feel able to ask more questions from a member of the team whom they find more approachable. Frequently the shock of the diagnosis prevents patients from taking in what is being said.

It is also possible, particularly if the outlook is not good, that patients will question different members of the team hoping to find a more optimistic prognosis. Clearly it is not in the patient's interest to hear conflicting opinions about their prognosis and this should be avoided.

Later, they may seek information from the internet which can be misleading. Openness regarding realistic treatment outcomes is also important in maintaining staff morale. While the death of a patient is often difficult, particularly for the nurses who are most closely involved in their care, this is especially so if unrealistic expectations of treatment have been fostered.

The goals of oncology treatment

Key Fact

Absolute and relative benefit of cancer treatment.

Absolute benefit relates to the benefit produced by undertaking a particular form of treatment.

Relative benefit relates to the benefit when compared to another form of treatment.

i.e. If the benefit of taking drug X instead of drug Y meant that ten year survival was increased from 5% to 7.5% this would indicate an absolute benefit of 2.5%, and a relative survival benefit of 50%.

Radical treatment

Radical oncological interventions are curative in intent. They may involve surgery, radiotherapy, chemotherapy, or a combination of these modalities.

Because the potential benefits of treatment are great, a relatively high incidence of toxicity is more acceptable.

Providing patients with good symptom control and emotional support throughout radical treatment is important. They need to be encouraged to complete what is often a very demanding treatment course to benefit maximally. Without such encouragement patients may miss the only opportunity they have of cure.

Increasingly, there is an appreciation that such treatments may be associated with long-term side effects. Clearly, in this potentially curable group, care must be taken to minimize the potential for cumulative dose toxicities such as cardiotoxicity caused by anthracyclines.

Adjuvant treatment

Many patients experience tumour relapse months or years after apparently curative surgery for their primary cancer. This is believed to be the result of the presence of micrometastatic disease that is not clinically apparent at the time of the primary treatment.

Anticancer treatment given after surgery when micrometastatic disease is suspected improves long-term survival for patients with some types of cancer such as breast and colon cancer.

This is true for tumours where chemotherapy would not be curative in the metastatic setting and is presumably related to the increased chemosensitivity associated with microscopic volumes of disease.

The absolute gains in survival from adjuvant therapy are generally modest but real. Adjuvant chemotherapy in premenopausal women with breast cancer for example is associated with an approximately 30% relative improvement in 10-year survival. At present there are few predictive factors to identify those patients most likely to benefit from adjuvant therapy. The decision to proceed is often based on the statistical likelihood of relapse, with those at highest risk generally having the most to gain.

Because the majority of patients will not benefit from adjuvant therapies, such treatments should have manageable acute toxicities and a low incidence of long-term complications.

Palliative treatment

Palliative treatment is indicated when cure is not possible but where treatments may improve cancer-related symptoms and can delay progression of disease or prolong survival. In many cases improvement of symptoms is accompanied by tumour shrinkage that is detectable clinically or by radiological methods such as CT scan or MRI. Increasingly, however, it is recognized that there may be a palliative benefit even in the absence of major tumour shrinkage.

As an important object of therapy is to maintain or improve quality of life, such treatments should be well tolerated with a low incidence of acute side effects. Long-term toxicities are generally not relevant.

Patients presenting with advanced ovarian cancer, for example, usually have incurable disease. However, the tumour is often chemosensitive and lengthy remissions are often seen following primary chemotherapy. In such patients a relatively high incidence of acute toxicity may be acceptable, with efforts being focused on managing chemotherapy-related symptoms. Conversely, a patient presenting with relapsed ovarian cancer soon after first-line chemotherapy has a low expectation of benefit from further chemotherapy. Consequently only a low incidence of acute toxicity is acceptable with second-line chemotherapy, from which expectation of benefit is very limited.

Clinical trials

Clinical research is necessary to improve outcome for patients with cancer. The link between the laboratory

---

Stop and Think

What does palliative mean?
The word *palliative* is used to mean different things to different people.

Palliative treatment from an oncologist will usually involve the use of oncological treatments aimed at prolonging survival and maintaining quality of life in patients who can no longer be offered curative treatment.

Palliative treatment from a palliative medicine specialist will focus on reducing disease-related symptoms (physical, emotional, and spiritual) in patients towards the end of their disease.

Palliative care may be understood by patients as meaning end of life care, whereas those receiving palliative radiotherapy or chemotherapy may survive for several years.

Test Yourself

Studies show that there are consistently improved outcomes for patients enrolled in clinical trials compared with patients who are not enrolled. Why might this be?

---

and the clinic is developing and increasingly patients are being recruited into trials.

There are three main types of clinical trial: Phase I, Phase II, and Phase III.

Phase I

Aims

◆ To establish the human toxicity of a new drug through delivering carefully selected increasing doses to patients

◆ To establish a safe dose at which to start further trials with the drug

◆ To evaluate the body's handling of the drug by pharmacokinetic studies

Eligible patients

Patients typically have progressive disease despite standard oncological therapy or tumours for which no standard therapy exists.

Small numbers of patients are used, i.e. 10–20. These patients must be aware that the primary objective of the studies is to assess tolerability and side effects. There is little expectation of benefit for themselves, with a response rate of approximately 5%.

Patients may have a range of tumour types but must have a good performance status. They also need to be highly motivated, since involvement often requires frequent visits to the hospital and additional investigations. Tissue biopsies and functional imaging studies may be used to demonstrate that the drug hits its intended molecular target.

Phase II

Aims

◆ To establish the activity (usually tumour shrinkage) of the drug against a particular tumour type

Eligible patients

Patients have a specific tumour, usually with progressive disease despite standard chemotherapy.

They usually require a good performance status and motivation.

Patients are closely monitored with toxicity and response assessments but not as intensively as those in Phase I studies.

Moderate numbers of patients are often required (50–200).

Phase III

Aim

◆ To compare the new treatment with conventional therapy

Eligible patients

Usually those for whom a standard therapy exists. New drugs may, however, be compared with 'best supportive care' where no standard therapy exists.

Large numbers of patients (hundreds or thousands) are often required to demonstrate clear benefit.

Important and common end points include overall survival (in adjuvant studies) and disease-free survival (in non-curative studies). Increasingly, more clinically relevant end points such as improvements in pain, performance status, weight gain, and quality of life are being used in Phase III trials of agents in the palliative setting or as secondary end points. However, patients require less intensive monitoring than in early trials.

End points

In any clinical trial it is vital to have defined the end points by which the trial will be judged at the outset. End points can be primary, relating to the central question of the trial, or secondary, relating to other outcomes such as side effects.

Survival

Survival is the ideal end point, but may require long follow-up, and the effect of the trial treatment may be obscured by subsequent therapy.

Disease-free survival

In the adjuvant disease-free survival is the length of time between initial treatment and recurrence of cancer. Time to progression is the time from treatment to progression of the cancer in patients with metastatic disease.

Test Yourself

Would you enter a Phase I clinical trial?

> **Key Facts**
>
> **The commonest end points used in clinical trials include:**
>
> ◆ Survival
>
> ◆ Disease-free survival
>
> ◆ Time to progression
>
> ◆ Response
>
> ◆ Toxicity
>
> ◆ Quality of life

Response

Response is a very useful end point in trials looking at new agents and their potential efficacy. There are clear definitions of response. One is the RECIST criteria based on the longest diameter of target lesion.

◆ Complete response (CR) – complete disappearance of all detectable disease for at least 1 month

◆ Partial response (PR) – ≥ 30% reduction in measurable disease for at least 1 month

◆ Stable disease (SD) – neither sufficient reduction to qualify as a PR nor sufficient increase to qualify as progressive disease

◆ Progressive disease (PD) – ≥ 20% increase in size of measurable disease during the treatment period

Before the commencement of the trial, clear measurement parameters will need to be defined, and it would be best if the measurement were carried out by independent observers.

Toxicity

These measures are crucial to ensure that the benefits of treatment clearly outweigh both short-term and long-term side effects. Assessment may be carried out using blood investigations as well as by scoring the severity of anticipated symptoms.

Quality of life

Quality of life measures look at the global impact of the trial treatment on the patient's life including side effects and psychological effects of the treatment.

Common examples used are the EORTC QLQ-C30 (European Organization for Research on Treatment of Cancer Quality of Life Questionnaire) and FACT (Functional Assessment of Cancer Treatment).

Chapter summary

- The early signs of cancer are often easier to see retrospectively than at their first appearance

- Cancer diagnosis and staging must be carried out in a systematic and thorough manner

- Improved imaging techniques have reduced the need for many major diagnostic surgical interventions

- Staging involves histological classification and defining the extent of the disease

- Goals of treatment need to be clear

- Radical treatment aims at cure and thus makes a high incidence of treatment toxicity acceptable

- Adjuvant treatment, usually chemotherapy given after surgery, aims to improve long-term survival

- Palliative treatment is aimed at prolonging survival and improving cancer-related symptoms when cure is no longer possible

- Clinical trials play a vital role in establishing whether a new treatment is safe and effective

- Before commencing any trial it is important to have determined clear end points and to stipulate how these end points will be measured

Communication with cancer patients

Introduction

Optimal care of the patient with cancer requires input from a number of medical disciplines. Typically, a provisional diagnosis of cancer is made by a surgeon or physician and confirmed by a pathologist following biopsy or fine-needle aspiration. A surgeon or an oncologist may then undertake definitive treatment. Support of the patient through treatment may well involve input from a wide range of surgical and medical staff as well as professions allied to medicine and laboratory disciplines.

Stop and Think

In what manner would you like to have bad news broken to you or your family?

Several factors facilitate this care:

- Good organization of cancer services
- Cancer site specialization for surgeons and oncologists
- Multidisciplinary team working
- Well-established links with laboratory and clinical cancer research
- A close working relationship between all health care professionals involved in the treatment. In the past, this relationship was not optimal because of misunderstandings of their different roles and treatment

Key Fact

The communication balance

There is a balance to be made between fully informing the patient about their disease and prognosis, completely overwhelming them with facts and figures, and providing only minimal and inadequate information.

While it is important to avoid being patronizing, it is also important not to cause 'information overload'.

aims. Increasingly, the goals are shared and closer working relationships are being forged, at different points in the patient's disease

◆ Oncological, diagnostic, medical, nursing, allied health professionals, specialist and generalist palliative care services, including the general practitioner and community health team, need to share information quickly so, at this point, when patient and family feel particularly vulnerable, informed support can be maximized[1]

Initial diagnosis

Receiving news that you have cancer is a shock even if it is not a surprise. Patients can often remember in intimate detail the day and hour they were given the information. A proportion of patients will find it impossible to concentrate on any other fact than 'I have cancer' and will be unable to take in much other information. While the news of cancer cannot be sugar coated, how the news is broken can have a profound effect on how a patient adapts to their disease and the treatments available. It is no longer acceptable for doctors to claim that breaking such news is not a skill that they possess, leaving it to others. Breaking bad news well is now regarded as a core skill that can be taught and increasingly patients are unforgiving of those who do it badly or insensitively.

'When I was diagnosed with my bowel cancer I was simply devastated. You see, I had watched my father dying from lung cancer and I was sure I would go the same way. I couldn't get out of the hospital quickly enough. The doctor said something about treatment, but I knew from watching others with cancer that treatment was pointless, so I never went back for the specialist appointment.

'It was only after my own doctor came out and we had a good chat that I even thought that they could do anything for me. In the end I decided to go and see what they were offering, still never believing that they could do any good.

'I honestly believe if my own doctor hadn't taken the time to come and explain that there really was something they could do to help I would not be here today.'

Through period of staging and/or surgery

This can be a time of great uncertainty for patients when communicating the often complex prognostic and treatment information is so important. Many find the issues very difficult to grasp, so major are the associated life implications. An understanding of these issues and of the likely treatments by all those involved in the clinical and supportive care of patient and family can help to consolidate information exchange. It is often only a few days after a crucial oncology outpatient appointment that patients become receptive to important information.

If other health care professionals are hesitant or contradictory in their explanations of treatment options, patient anxiety will be increased.

Through period of treatment

While the majority of supportive care during this period tends to be linked through the oncology services, all professionals involved with providing the treatment and supportive care may benefit from sharing information at a case conference highlighting the:

◆ Goals of treatment

◆ The side effects of treatment

◆ Follow-up plans

At point of relapse

This is usually a very difficult time for patients when their fears are confirmed that their disease is no longer being controlled by oncological treatments. Many patients focus on 'being positive' to the extent that they outwardly deny any possibility of the disease not being cured by treatment. Being told that the disease has relapsed can seem overwhelming. In addition, if treatment strategies are being changed from curative to palliative, with much less intervention, patients can easily feel abandoned by the oncological team.

At point of dying

Honesty and support for patients and their families are often crucial at this point, ensuring that opportunities for communication and spiritual support, where wanted, are maximized.

Communicating with patients undergoing oncology treatments

Chemotherapy and radiotherapy are now given largely on an outpatient basis. Surgical patients also spend less time in hospital than in the past. This allows patients to spend more time at home, but inevitably places an increased burden of care on those providing support in the community, particularly where the cancer centre is a long distance from home. Thus a general understanding of the particular side effects, and the appropriate treatment for such complications, is needed increasingly by health care professionals in the community and by those providing on-call services.

Breaking bad news

- Patients and relatives need time to absorb information and to adapt to bad news

- Health professionals need good communication skills, including sensitivity and empathic active listening

- Breaking bad news takes time and issues often need to be discussed further and clarified as more information is imparted

There is increasing evidence that most patients want to know about their illness. Many patients who have been denied this knowledge have difficulty in understanding why they are becoming weaker and are then relieved and grateful to be told the truth. Patients may be angry with the family who have known about the illness all along and have not thought it right to tell them.

As professionals, we may become entangled in a 'conspiracy of silence' situation when the family demands information before we have had a chance to speak to the patient. They might say, 'Do not tell him the diagnosis/prognosis because he would not be able to cope with it. We know him better than you do.' This can be an awkward situation. The family need to know

that we have understood their concerns of not wanting to cause any more hurt to the patient. They also need to know that we accept that some patients use denial as a way of coping. However, they also need to know that it would be unwise for clinical staff to be untruthful if the patient appeared to want to know the truth and was asking direct questions, because of the inevitable breakdown in trust that this could cause.

Prognostication

Advising patients and families with regard to prognosis is important since they may want to try to organize their affairs and plan for the time that is left, but, **it is impossible to be accurate**. Overestimating or underestimating the time that someone has to live can cause untold anguish. It is therefore more sensible to talk in terms of days/weeks, weeks/months, and months/years as appropriate.

It is important to be aware that people have differing attitudes to receiving bad news and that this needs sensitive handling. Furthermore, people respond badly to being told bad news in a hurried, brusque and unsympathetic manner with no time to collect thoughts and ask questions.

A strategy for breaking bad news

This strategy outlines what other people have found helpful. Individuals should develop their personal ways of breaking bad news based on these principles. Practice and critical self-reflection are necessary to continue to improve this basic but essential skill.

The goals of breaking bad news

The process of breaking bad news needs to be specifically tailored to the needs of the individual concerned because every human being will have a different history and collection of fears and concerns.

The goal of breaking bad news is to do so in a way that facilitates acceptance and understanding and reduces the risk of destructive responses.

Preparing to tell bad news

Acquire all the information possible about the patient and their family. A 'genogram' (family tree) is particularly useful in quickly assimilating the important people in the patient's life, and the web of relationships within the family.

Read the patient's notes for:

- Diagnostic information
- Test results

Test Yourself

When is bad news about cancer most likely to be broken?
The commonest scenarios for breaking bad news to patients with cancer are at diagnosis, at the point of relapse or progression, or at the beginning of terminal care.

- Full details of the patient's clinical history

- The support system for the individual

- Background knowledge of the patient's life. Making basic mistakes will undermine the patient's confidence

Discuss with other members of the team, and then select the most appropriate team member to break the bad news.

Decide which other member of the team should be present during the interview.

Check the following:

- Private place with tissues, jug of water and glasses

- Time to carry out process

- Your own emotional energy to do so (better earlier in the day than later)

- Pressing tasks are completed so that there will be minimal interruptions – unplug the telephone and switch off the mobile phone etc.

Let the patient speak first

Avoid closed questions (ones that lead to 'yes'/'no' answers) in favour of open questions, such as:-

'How are you feeling today?'

'Can you tell me how this all came about?'

'How do you see things going from here?"

Plan

Prepare a rough plan in your mind of what you want to achieve in the communication, and what you want to avoid communicating. Having a rough goal will bring structure to the communication, though it is important to avoid imposing your agenda on the patient's agenda.

Set the context

Introduce yourself clearly.

Let the patient know they have your undivided attention. Ensure that the patient is comfortable and not distracted by pain or a full bladder etc.

Give 'warning shot' indication that this is not a social or routine encounter.

Key Fact

A 'warning shot' is concerned with preparing a patient that bad news is coming. This allows them to be more receptive than if it comes 'out of the blue'.

An example would be, 'I'm sorry to say that the results were not as good as we had hoped.'

Stop and Think

Sympathy = feeling another's pain.

Empathy = understanding another's pain.

Sit at the same level as the patient within easy reach and not behind an obstacle such as a desk.

Assess

- How much the patient knows already

- How much the patient wants to know. 'Are you the sort of person who likes to know everything?'

- How the patient expresses themselves verbally and non-verbally

- What words and ways of understanding their situation they use

Show empathy with the patient

- What would it be like to be the patient?

- How is the patient feeling?

- Is there anything that is concerning the patient?

- What mechanisms has the patient used in the past to deal with bad news?

- Does the patient have a particular outlook on life or cultural understanding?

- Who are the important people in the patient's life?

Respond to **non-verbal** as well as **verbal** cues.

Encourage the patient to speak by listening carefully, not interrupting, and responding appropriately.

Ten steps to breaking bad news (adapted from Kaye, 1996[2])

1 **Preparation**

Know all the facts before the meeting. READ THE NOTES! Find out who the patient wants to be present. Ensure comfort and privacy. Minimize the risks of interruptions

2 **What does the patient know?**

Ask the patient for a brief narrative of events (e.g. how did it all start?)

3 **Give a warning shot**

e.g. 'I am afraid it looks rather serious' – then allow a pause for the patient to respond

4 **Allow denial**

Allow the patient to control the amount of information and to proceed at their own pace

5 **Explain (if requested) and check understanding**
Narrow the information gap step by step. Use diagrams if the patient thinks they would be helpful. Use appropriate language

6 **Is more information wanted?**
It can be very frightening to ask for more information and patients may not want to know any more! Test the waters by asking e.g. 'would you like me to explain a bit more?'

7 **Listen to concerns**
Ask, 'What are the things that bother you most at the moment?' This could be to do with physical or emotional health or relate to social or spiritual issues

8 **Encourage ventilation of feelings**
This conveys empathy and may be the key phase in terms of patient satisfaction with the interview. Check that there is nothing else that they want to talk about

9 **Summary and plan**
Summarize concerns, plan treatment and foster hope. Check with the patient that they would have no objection for you to talk with the family either alone or with the patient

10 **Offer availability**
Most patients need further explanation (the details will not have been remembered) and support (adjustment takes weeks or months) and benefit greatly from a family meeting. In addition, written material or a recording of the interview may be a useful adjunct to good communication

---

Key Facts

◆ Listen to patients

◆ Be honest, but not brutal

◆ Repeat information and check understanding

◆ Let the patient know there is a plan whatever the situation

---

Chapter summary

◆ Many professionals are involved in the care of patients with cancer so clear communication is vital, particularly at the time of diagnosis or when there is a sudden change in management

◆ Patient anxiety will be increased by conflicting information

◆ No single health professional can manage the many needs which patients have on their cancer journey

◆ It is good practice to inform other key health workers in the care of the patient on the details of crucial conversations, especially those where bad news has been broken

References

1. National Council for Hospice and Specialist Palliative Care Services. *Definition of supportive and palliative care*. (Briefing Bulletin 11). London: NCHSPCS, 2002,

2. Kaye P. *Breaking bad news*. Northampton: E.P.L. Publications, 1996.

Oncological surgery

Surgery remains the modality of treatment most likely to cure patients diagnosed with solid tumours.[1] It has most potential when the cancer is localized, though results are also significantly improving for patients with certain types of metastatic tumours.

Surgery has three main roles in cancer management:

- Diagnosis and staging
- Curative treatment
- Palliative treatment

Diagnosis and staging

In the past, many patients suspected of having cancer required surgery to confirm the diagnosis. The ability to perform diagnostic biopsies using radiological guidance or endoscopy now often permit accurate diagnosis without recourse to open surgery.

Patient morbidity is significantly reduced now that major diagnostic surgical procedures are often no longer needed and radiological staging is much improved. The number of 'open and close' laparotomies for unresectable cancer, for example, has fallen to < 5% in recent years largely because of advances in imaging and laparoscopic techniques.

However, surgical staging remains important in a number of common tumours.

Axillary lymph node dissection for patients with breast cancer allows assessment of these nodes for tumour involvement. Such information is important in determining prognosis and guiding decisions regarding adjuvant treatments.

Ovarian cancer spreads mainly via the transperitoneal route leading to tumour deposits on peritoneal surfaces and the omentum – sites poorly visualized on conventional imaging. A **laparotomy** for patients with ovarian cancer therefore allows more accurate staging of disease than is currently possible with non-invasive means. Again such information is vital in determining prognosis and guiding further treatment. Laparoscopy in certain abdominal malignancies is a useful staging tool before a major resection.

Key Facts

Sentinel lymph node assessment (used particularly for breast cancer and melanoma)

♦ The sentinel lymph node is the node which will usually first receive tumour cells from the tumour site

♦ Methylene blue dye and a radioisotope injected preoperatively allows the node to be identified during surgery and removed for histological examination

♦ If negative for tumour a radical lymph node dissection, with its associated morbidity, may be avoided

♦ Detailed histological examination of the sentinel node often shows micrometastases but their clinical implication in terms of prognosis and treatment is uncertain

---

Curative surgery

Non-metastatic disease

Surgery is most commonly curative in intent for localized cancers and is generally dependent on complete resection of the tumour with a margin of normal tissue.

In some tumours with a propensity to spread to lymph nodes, resection of the draining lymph nodes may improve local control (e.g. vulval tumours). En bloc removal of the immediate lymphatic drainage area is usually a major goal of cancer surgery. In other tumours the value of lymphadenectomy is uncertain and is the subject of ongoing clinical trials (e.g. endometrial cancer).

Unfortunately, surgery still fails to cure many patients whose cancer returns at a later date despite having appeared to be completely removed at operation. There are a number of reasons for this:

♦ Development of metastatic disease – this is the result of the presence of **micrometastatic disease** that could not be detected at the time of surgery. This is a common reason for failure of surgery to cure breast and bowel tumours

♦ Development of local relapse – outcomes from surgery are often closely linked to the margin of normal tissue excised in continuity with the tumour. The amount of tissue that can be resected may be limited by patient-related factors (e.g. only a partial lobectomy may be possible in patients with lung cancer because of the patients' underlying poor respiratory function) or by tumour-related factors (e.g. invasion by tumour of a vital structure such as the aorta)

Metastatic disease

Although much less common, surgery may be curative in a limited number of tumours with metastases. These include:

♦ Pulmonary metastases from osteosarcoma or soft tissue sarcoma

♦ Residual masses following chemotherapy for metastatic teratomas

♦ Liver metastases from colorectal cancer

In each of these cases best results are seen with careful patient selection according to well-defined criteria after multidisciplinary assessment. Surgery by a specialist team is usually best.

Test Yourself

Which patients do best with surgery for metastatic cancer?
In general terms the best long-term results from surgery for metastatic cancer are seen in patients who relapse a long time after the initial tumour diagnosis, who have low volume disease and a good performance status.

Palliative surgery

Surgery may provide very effective palliation in a number of situations. Given the specific problems of oncology patients in the palliative setting (limited life expectancy, poor performance status, rapid tumour progression), the decision to proceed with surgery must involve a careful weighing up of the benefit/harm of such procedures. These decisions are best made with a multidisciplinary approach including surgeons specialized in oncology.

Bowel obstruction

Patients with colonic or ovarian cancer form the majority of patients with bowel obstruction referred for surgery. Surgery to relieve the obstruction may be warranted even if disease is incurable (due to liver metastases or locally advanced disease for example) as such patients may live for many months. Patients with colorectal cancer may present with bowel obstruction, with or without metastatic disease. Where possible these patients should have the primary tumour excised and a primary anastomosis performed. Endoscopic stent insertion may help selected patients.

Patients with ovarian cancer may also present with obstructive bowel symptoms. At initial presentation debulking surgery provides excellent palliation. Patients presenting with relapsed disease and obstructive symptoms often have multiple sites of obstruction because of widespread intraperitoneal dissemination of their disease. In this situation surgery is less likely to be useful.

Fistulae

Fistulae may arise as a result of pelvic tumours or as a complication of radiotherapy.

They are often associated with unpleasant symptoms such as discharge of faeces from the vagina. Optimal preoperative assessment requires imaging to delineate exactly the site of fistula formation and to guide surgical decisions.

Surgery may provide excellent palliation but may not be useful in those with multiple sites of fistula or rapidly advancing intra-abdominal disease where life expectancy is limited. This is difficult, complex surgery.

Jaundice

Obstructive jaundice as a result of extrinsic pressure by lymph nodes on the biliary system or intrinsic lesions such as cholangiocarcinoma or pancreatic carcinoma

are commonly well palliated by radiological and endoscopic placement of stents.

The complications of stents include infection and blockage with the consequent need for replacement.

Surgical relief of obstructive jaundice (e.g. by choledochoenterostomy) avoids the problems associated with stents and may be indicated in a small minority of patients with an excellent performance status and slowly growing disease.

Spinal cord compression and brain tumours

In situations when patients have confirmed spinal cord compression or isolated brain metastases, urgent referral for neurosurgical assessment for decompressive surgery is usually the management option of choice.

Gastrointestinal bleeding

A wide range of endoscopic techniques have been developed to stop bleeding from benign and malignant causes. This may avoid the need for major surgery in patients who have a limited life expectancy.

These include:

◆ Sclerotherapy with adrenaline

◆ Laser coagulation

◆ Radiological embolization

Bone metastases

Metastases to bones can cause major palliation problems. Specific problems include pain and pathological fracture. Factors that identify patients most at risk of pathological fracture include:

◆ Site – lesions in weight-bearing bones

◆ Extent of destruction – destruction of > 50% of cortex

◆ Symptoms – patients complaining of pain particularly on weight bearing

◆ Type of lesion – lytic lesions more than blastic lesions

Such patients may benefit (both in terms of reduced pain and reduced risk of fracture) from prophylactic fixation of a long bone. The type of internal fixation used depends on the site of the metastasis, the patient's performance status, and life expectancy.

In all cases internal fixation of the bone should be followed by radiotherapy to control tumour growth and promote healing.

Techniques such as vertebroplasty are available to manage pain in the vertebrae.

Key Facts

Palliation of obstructive symptoms
Nephrostomy or ureteric catheters may relieve obstructive hydronephrosis.

Laser therapy of an intraluminal mass may restore the lumen of an obstructed oesophagus or bronchus.

Placement of a stent may overcome the symptoms of:

◆ Dysphagia (oesophagus)

◆ Dyspnoea (bronchus)

◆ Large bowel obstruction (colon)

Pain

Surgical debulking of large, slowly growing tumours can reduce pain and is justified in patients where the expected morbidity of the procedure is low.

Neurosurgical approaches such as cordotomy (cutting the pain fibres in the spinal cord) are only rarely considered.

Some surgeons will carry out an 'open' coeliac axis block during surgery for upper gastrointestinal malignancies, where painful local invasion can be anticipated but this is less necessary with modern pain management.

Test Yourself

Mrs White has advanced breast carcinoma, with widespread bone metastases. Today she fell at home and sustained a pathological fracture of her right hip. How would you determine if it were appropriate to refer her for internal fixation?

Combined surgery and radiotherapy (and in some cases chemotherapy) are used in specific circumstances

Benefits

- In instances of rectal cancers where the tumour is large or starting to invade adjacent tissues, combining radiotherapy with surgery may achieve better local control rates than using either treatment modality on its own
- Radiotherapy supports surgery by treating microscopic disease sites adjacent to the area of surgery
- Pre-operative radiotherapy may make surgery easier by shrinking the tumour bulk

Problems

- Healing rates may be slowed by pre-operative radiotherapy
- Histological clarity may be lost by pre-operative radiotherapy because biopsies may be difficult to interpret
- Logistical problems can be magnified by the involvement of two very busy clinical services with a delay in one or other treatment modality

Reference

1. Cassidy J, *et al. Oxford Handbook of Oncology*. Oxford: Oxford University Press, 2002.

Key Facts

Pre-operative therapy = neoadjuvant therapy.

Post-operative therapy = adjuvant therapy,

Chapter summary

- Surgery remains the modality of treatment most likely to cure patients with localized disease
- Patient morbidity has been significantly reduced through less invasive diagnostic procedures
- Localized cancers have the greatest chance of cure with surgery

Although much less common, surgery may be curative in a limited number of tumours in the metastatic setting. These include:

- Pulmonary metastases from osteosarcoma or soft tissue sarcoma
- Liver metastases from colorectal cancer
- Residual masses following chemotherapy for metastatic teratomas

Surgery may provide very effective palliation in a number of situations:

- Bowel obstruction
- Fistulae
- Jaundice
- Gastrointestinal bleeding
- Spinal cord compression and brain tumours
- Bone metastases
- Pain

CHAPTER 6

Systemic therapy: chemotherapy and biological therapy

'Regardless of one victory, two victories, four victories, there's never been a victory by a cancer survivor. That's a fact that hopefully I'll be remembered for.'

Lance Edward Armstrong (1971–),
Winner of seven consecutive Tour de France races
(1999–2005)

Treatment of localized disease with surgery or radiotherapy can be very effective, but most deaths from cancer are the result of metastatic disease. Systemic therapy (i.e. drugs that can treat cancer wherever it may be in the body) are therefore vitally important. Chemotherapy drugs that 'poison' cancer cells remain the most widely used systemic therapies, but new targeted biological therapies are becoming increasingly important.

Chemotherapy still provokes strong but often misguided or inaccurate reactions from sections of the public. Such reactions are easily accessible on the internet, and many of our patients will have been exposed to such views prior to attending the clinic. Others will have spoken to friends or relatives whose experience of chemotherapy comes from a different era and refers to different drugs, used to treat different types of cancer and with different methods of reducing drug side effects.

Introduction

Chemotherapy generally refers to a group of 'cytotoxic' agents used in the systemic management of cancer. A disparate group, they are linked by having demonstrated evidence of anti-cancer activity and a common range of side effects. They are important because very often cancer is a systemic, rather than a localized, disease.

The smallest clinically detectable tumour lump is approximately 1 cm in diameter and already contains one billion tumour cells. Therefore, the potential to develop secondary tumours and metastatic disease at distant sites throughout the body is significant, even in the earliest detectable lesion.

Patients usually do not die as a result of local recurrence in the primary organ but as a result of systemic spread of the disease. Therefore, treatment to eradicate occult cancer cells must include effective systemic treatment. Today, approximately 60–70% of cancer patients will require chemotherapy as part of the treatment of their disease.

Identification of agents

The anti-cancer activity of chemotherapy agents has been identified in different ways.

For some agents the discovery of their antineoplastic activity was by chance. Cisplatin was discovered because platinum electrodes were toxic in an antibiotic experiment.

For other agents this activity was identified during the purposeful screening of a wide range of natural products (e.g. paclitaxel).

Some are analogues to existing cytotoxics that have been biochemically modified either to reduce their toxicity or to increase their antineoplastic activity (e.g. carboplatin was derived from cisplatin).

Mechanism of action

Chemotherapy exerts its anti-cancer action by a wide variety of mechanisms which are, as yet, incompletely understood although most target DNA either directly or indirectly. Chemotherapeutic agents are preferentially toxic towards actively proliferating cells.

Test Yourself

How would you advise a patient with cancer who has the potential to be cured by chemotherapy but is reluctant to embark on treatment?

Stop and Think

Chemotherapy has cured thousands of patients and prolonged and improved the quality of life of many more, so why does it provoke such strong reactions?

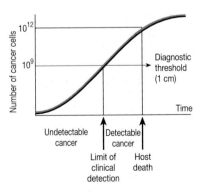

Fig. 6.1 Growth of cancer cells over time.

Key Fact

Tumours which divide rapidly with short doubling times usually respond best to chemotherapy.

The various phases that make up the proliferating phases of the cell cycle are termed G_1, S, G_2, and M; the resting phase is termed G_0.

G_1 = Protein synthesis phase
S = DNA synthesis
G_2/M = cellular division
G_0 = resting phase

Chemotherapy drugs may affect different phases of the cell cycle.

A number of factors determine the likelihood of achieving a useful response to chemotherapy.

Some tumours are inherently more sensitive to chemotherapy than others. In general terms, chemotherapy tends to be most effective in tumours with fast cell turnover such as acute leukaemias and high-grade lymphomas. However, seminomas, which have a long natural history, are also very chemosensitive. Clearly there are other factors, as yet poorly understood, that determine a tumour's chemosensitivity. In particular, it appears that although cytotoxic drugs consistently cause DNA damage, tumour cells differ with regard to their response (death or recovery) to that damage.

Combining different chemotherapy agents may increase the potential to improve outcomes

- Using agents with different mechanisms of action increases tumour cell destruction
- Combining agents with non-overlapping toxicities permits the administration of close to full doses of two or more active agents at once

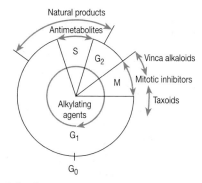

Fig. 6.2 Cell cycle.

- In practice, most chemotherapy combinations have been developed empirically
- Sequential use of individual agents may be as effective as combination therapy

Chemotherapy dose intensity

The total dose of chemotherapy and the overall treatment time are two variables that have a significant impact on the effectiveness of a given drug treatment. Realization of this has led to the evaluation of dose intensity (total amount of chemotherapy/unit time) of various treatment schedules and suggested the concept that high dose intensity is beneficial. In general, substantially reducing the dose intensity reduces the efficacy of treatment. For most cancers it is unclear, however, if increasing the dose intensity significantly improves outcome.

Chemotherapy cure

The probability of cure with chemotherapy is inversely proportional to the tumour burden for the following reasons:

- The greater the tumour burden the greater the likelihood of resistance developing
- The greater the tumour burden the smaller the growth fraction
- The greater the tumour burden the higher the probability of metastatic spread

Patient-related factors are also important in determining the likelihood of response. Patients with poor performance status, for example, respond less well than those who are fitter. The reasons for this are poorly understood but are probably, at least partly, the result of a reduced tolerance to the acute toxicity of chemotherapy.

Chemoresistance

Some cancers are resistant to chemotherapy from the outset. For others, chemotherapy may induce a partial or even complete response but the tumour regrows with disease that has become chemoresistant. Increasingly it is recognized that the ability of cells to either repair or tolerate the damage inflicted by chemotherapy may lead to chemoresistance.

An A to Z of adverse effects of chemotherapy

Cytotoxic chemotherapy often causes significant toxicity. In part, this is because, to be effective, cytotoxics must be administered at a dose close to the maximum

TABLE 6.1	Mechanisms of drug resistance	
Mechanism	**Drug**	**Effect**
Multidrug resistance	Anthracyclines	Increased drug efflux through active transport
	Vinca alkaloids	
	Etoposide	
	Taxanes	
Impaired transport	Methotrexate	
	Melphalan	Decreased binding sites or carrier activity
Impaired drug activation	Cytarabine	Low cytidine kinase
	Methotrexate	Low polyglutamation
Increased inactivation	Cytarabine	High cytidine deaminase
	Alkylating agents	Increased glutathione and cellular thiols
Improved DNA repair	Platinum compounds	Increased excision of damaged DNA
Target alterations	Methotrexate	Increased levels of dihydrofolate reductase, or mutations in the enzyme
	5-Fluorouracil	Altered levels of activity of thymidylate synthase

that can safely be given. Unlike most other drugs, if cytotoxics were given at half the standard dose, they would usually be ineffective and, if given at twice the normal dose, they may well be lethal.

Alopecia

This is a common and often distressing side effect associated with many agents. Patients can be reassured that hair almost always regrows following chemotherapy although they may notice some changes. The hair may change colour and change in 'curliness'. The use of a 'cold cap' to protect hair follicles is used in some centres with some drugs to decrease the extent of alopecia. The cap is put on 15 minutes before chemotherapy to start restricting the blood flow, and is kept on during and up to 1–2 hours after the chemotherapy. This technique does not prevent alopecia after high dose chemotherapy.

Anxiety

The prospect of chemotherapy is frightening for many patients – not least because of the (often mistaken) view of the difficult side effects. It is important that the patients and their carers are fully educated about the type of side effects they are likely to encounter during

treatment and how best to deal with them. Most patients are extremely anxious during this difficult time and information may have to be repeated a number of times. It is very useful to have written information to supplement what has been said in consultations. It also useful if a relative or friend attends with the patient – they will often be able to help the patient review the information at a later date.

Cardiotoxicity

This has been associated in particular with anthracyclines such as doxorubicin and daunorubicin. There may be transient cardiomyopathy with congestive heart failure, particularly when the cumulative dose of doxorubicin approaches 450–550 mg/m^2. Chest radiotherapy may also lead to cardiotoxicity and constrictive pericarditis.

Fatigue

Perhaps the commonest side effect of chemotherapy, fatigue, can vary in intensity from just feeling a little less energetic to such an experience of overwhelming weariness that patients may describe it as a constant ache. Treatment is available in terms of lifestyle modification, medication, and the treatment of contributory factors such as anaemia or depression. Encouraging patients to keep as active as possible within the confines of their weakness is important. Advances in the management of fatigue over the next few years may produce significant improvements in reducing the substantial morbidity associated with fatigue.

Gonadal damage and sterility

Several drugs, including the alkylating agents or others such as vinblastine, procarbazine, and the cytosine analogues, may lead to sterility in both men and women. For young men receiving these drugs it is wise to consider sperm storage. The role of egg harvesting in women is not as clear.

Immunosuppression

While patients are on chemotherapy, one must assume that they are immunosuppressed, and therefore susceptible to infections.

Myelosuppression

The white cells (in particular the neutrophils) are most commonly affected between 1 and 2 weeks following chemotherapy. Patients should be warned of the possibility of developing infection during this time and told of the importance of seeking help urgently because they may require immediate treatment with broad spectrum intravenous antibiotics. The development of granulocyte colony-stimulating growth factors has reduced this toxicity by shortening the duration of neutropenia. This has allowed higher doses of chemotherapy to be given more safely in certain situations and is used in neutropenic sepsis.

Nausea and vomiting

These are common with many agents, although, with modern antiemetics, emesis is now much less of a problem. The degree to which this is a problem varies both between agents and between patients. The development of $5HT_3$ (serotonin) antagonists (e.g. tropisetron, granisetron) has greatly aided the management of this troublesome side effect. The efficacy of $5HT_3$ antagonists is improved by the addition of steroids.

Neurotoxicity

Neurotoxicity is most commonly associated with vincristine, cisplatin, oxaliplatin and paclitaxel. These drugs cause peripheral neuropathy characterized by loss of deep tendon reflexes, paraesthesia, motor weakness, and occasional jaw or other pain. Procarbazine and L-asparagine, used in the treatment of leukaemia and lymphoma, may cause central nervous system symptoms including hallucinations and depression.

Ifosfamide may lead to the development of encephalopathy, which is usually reversible, but may lead to residual neurological side effects such as memory loss or drowsiness.

Pulmonary toxicity

Bleomycin is associated with pulmonary toxicity; it causes a decrease in diffusion capacity and total lung capacity. This occurs in approximately 10–15% of patients who receive bleomycin. Such fibrosis is usually only associated with doses of 300–350 units/m². However, it may also occur at lower doses and may be irreversible even when the drug is stopped.

Renal toxicity

Renal tubular necrosis can result from the use of agents such as cisplatin or methotrexate. Very occasionally these side effects are not reversible and patients will require dialysis.

Chemotherapy regimens

A wide and somewhat bewildering number of chemotherapy regimens are used in the treatment of patients with cancer. In general terms the tendency has been to combine drugs that demonstrate activity as single agents but which do not share the same side effects.

Chemotherapy is typically administered in 'cycles', repeated every 2–4 weeks once the side effects of previous treatment have resolved. If a patient experiences serious or life-threatening toxicity, the dose may be reduced in subsequent cycles or treatment even stopped. Where there is visible cancer (clinically or radiologically) the response to treatment is monitored every 2–3 cycles. If there is evidence of response (i.e. a reduction in the tumour mass) treatment continues typically for about 4 months (or six cycles of a 3-weekly regimen). If there is evidence of disease progression, the current regimen is usually discontinued; there would then be a discussion with the patient regarding further treatment options.

Chemotherapy may be given with two intentions (curative, palliative) in three settings (neoadjuvant, adjuvant, metastatic).

Chemotherapy – curative intention
Metastatic setting

A small number of solid malignancies are curable by chemotherapy alone. Such tumours include germ cell tumours, lymphomas, and certain childhood tumours.

In general terms, chemotherapy regimens used in the treatment of these diseases are intensive and associated with a high incidence of acute toxicity. It is important that patients receive chemotherapy on schedule, with no delays, as there is evidence that dose reductions and prolonged treatment times may adversely affect outcome. Consequently treatment can exact a high physical and psychological toll on patients and their relatives.

Given that the long-term aim of treatment is cure, patients and their carers need encouragement to persevere, which will be easier if physical symptoms are optimally managed. The palliative care team, for example, advise on control of chemotherapy-induced vomiting even when the intention remains cure.

Increasingly it is becoming clear that patients cured by chemotherapy are at risk of long-term toxicity arising from their treatment. Such problems include secondary leukaemias and solid tumours, fatigue, infertility, and cardiomyopathy. Undoubtedly as more people become long-term survivors of cancer, more problems will emerge. For this reason it is may be important that long-term survivors of cancer remain on indefinite follow-up instead of being discharged.

Adjuvant setting

This is the commonest form of curative chemotherapy. Many patients presenting with apparently localized cancer are at high risk of later developing metastatic disease. This is presumed to be because of the presence of micrometastases that are not apparent using the currently available imaging modalities. Chemotherapy given following successful primary local treatment may reduce the risk of patients developing clinical metastatic disease.

Cancers in which adjuvant chemotherapy is commonly used include breast and colorectal cancer where large multi-centre randomized controlled trials and subsequent meta-analysis have confirmed a survival benefit.

At an individual level these gains are modest with absolute improvements in overall survival of 5–15% after 5 years. At a population level however, this represents a large number of lives saved in diseases as common as breast and bowel cancer.

At present pathological features such as tumour size, tumour grade, and lymph node involvement are commonly used to assess the risk of disease relapse and thereby identify those patients most likely to benefit from adjuvant therapy. Much current research is directed towards developing predictive markers to identify more precisely those most likely to benefit.

Given that many patients treated with adjuvant chemotherapy will not benefit from treatment (either because their disease will still relapse, or they have already been completely cured by primary treatment), adjuvant regimens should be well tolerated with a low incidence of serious acute complications and long-term side effects.

Again, as with treatment in the curative setting, positive outcomes from treatment are closely linked to maintaining dose intensity and avoiding delays in chemotherapy.

Neoadjuvant setting

Chemotherapy may be used 'up front' before definitive treatment (usually surgery) for the primary tumour. This may be carried out in the case of a large inoperable primary tumour to shrink the cancer and facilitate surgery. Such an approach is standard practice for example in very large primary breast tumours or in those with skin involvement.

Increasingly, neoadjuvant therapy is also being utilized for tumours that are operable. Potential advantages of this approach include less extensive surgery for a tumour that has shrunk. In terms of understanding better the treatment of cancer, neoadjuvant treatment with biopsies before and after therapy may allow molecular markers that predict chemosensitivity to be identified.

Conversely there are a number of potential problems with neoadjuvant chemotherapy.

* There may be a loss of potentially useful prognostic information after chemotherapy when, for example, the axillary node status or size of a breast cancer has changed

* There is also the risk that such an approach may allow tumour progression if the tumour does not respond to chemotherapy

* Performing less radical surgery in a tumour that has responded to chemotherapy may compromise local control

This approach is being examined in a number of malignancies including oesophageal, gastric, and breast tumours.

Chemotherapy – palliative intention

The majority of adult solid cancers with clinically or radiologically visible metastases are not curable. Chemotherapy, however, may have a valuable role to play in the palliative treatment of such patients. Increasingly, clinical trials include end points such as quality of life and toxicity which are clinically relevant in this setting in addition to overall survival .

A patient may be best managed when chemotherapy is administered *in conjunction with* input from the palliative care team. Such input also facilitates the gradual handing over of care to the palliative care team

---

Stop and Think

'Growth for the sake of growth is the ideology of the cancer cell.'

Edward Abbey 1927–1989

Key Facts

Given that improvement or maintenance of quality of life is the most important aim of palliative chemotherapy, acute toxicities must be infrequent and easily managed.

if the patient's disease progresses. Such a team-based approach reduces the problems of a patient feeling abandoned by their oncologist when chemotherapy is no longer useful. Administering palliative chemotherapy whilst a patient is still relatively fit may maximize the chance of maintaining the patient's quality of life and mean that the disease will remain controlled for longer.

Selection of patients suitable for chemotherapy

The decision to use chemotherapy is often a complex matter and a number of factors must be taken into consideration.

Patient choice

Explaining the benefits and risks of chemotherapy to patients and their families requires good communication skills, time, and an up-to-date knowledge base. While a small proportion of patients will choose not to be involved in the decision-making process, the vast majority will, and it is essential that this work of information sharing is carried out well so that patients can make educated choices about treatment options.

Patient fitness

Generally, patients with Eastern Cooperative Oncology Group (ECOG) performance status > 2 tolerate chemotherapy very poorly; in most circumstances chemotherapy is not appropriate in such patients.

Possible exceptions include patients with very chemosensitive tumours that may be expected to respond quickly such as small cell lung cancer and lymphoma.

In addition medical conditions such as long-standing renal or cardiac problems may prevent certain chemotherapy regimens being appropriate for particular patients. Further, the psychological state of patients may make certain particularly stressful regimens ill-advised.

Treatment intent

If the patient's tumour is potentially curable and should respond to chemotherapy, the threshold to treat will be much lower than if the disease is poorly responsive to chemotherapy.

> **Test Yourself**
>
> **What are the indications for palliative chemotherapy?**
>
> 1) **Maintaining or improving quality of life:**
> This is the single most important aim of palliative chemotherapy.
>
> Chemotherapy may alleviate specific symptoms such as dyspnoea or chest pain in a patient with lung cancer. It may also improve or maintain general well-being with improvements in such factors as appetite and energy.
>
> The development of quality of life assessment tools, and especially those with disease-specific elements, has made it easier to assess the effect of chemotherapy on quality of life.
>
> 2) **Improving survival:**
> While it is a secondary objective in most cases, chemotherapy given with palliative intent frequently prolongs survival. The extent to which it is expected that survival may be prolonged varies between diseases. Chemotherapy in pancreatic cancer is associated with an improvement in survival of only a few weeks whereas patients receiving chemotherapy for ovarian cancer may have improved survival of many months or even years.
>
> 3) **In emergency situations:**
> Potentially life-threatening tumour-related emergencies such as spinal cord compression or superior vena caval obstruction may be treated with chemotherapy where the primary tumour is very chemosensitive. Such tumours include lymphoma and small cell lung cancer.

Disease sites

Generally large-volume disease at life-threatening sites such as the liver requires urgent chemotherapy even in the absence of disease-related symptoms, because patients are likely to become symptomatic very quickly.

Patient symptoms

Chemotherapy in the palliative setting is sometimes delayed until the patient develops symptoms. The potential danger with this approach is that the patient may rapidly develop symptoms which render them unfit for chemotherapy. In some cases, therefore, oncologists may choose to monitor disease and institute treatment when there is evidence that disease, although asymptomatic, is progressing.

Stop and Think

Close relationships may build up between oncologists and patients over many years. It may be
difficult for doctors to withdraw potentially toxic
and ineffective oncological treatment from a patient who continues to demand it even when it
becomes clearly inappropriate. Open discussion
with patients and their family about the potential
benefits and risks of chemotherapy, the aims of
treatment and, in particular, criteria for stopping
treatment is important.

How will chemotherapy affect the patient and family?

Each individual patient and family will have their own
particular response to chemotherapy. Certain themes
may be common to many individuals. The following
are some of the scenarios encountered in GP surgeries,
oncology services, and palliative care units.

'I'll try anything'

Having endured the rigours of their disease and its management some patients reach the chemotherapy clinic
protesting their capacity as 'fighters'. There is now evidence that psychological disposition has limited bearing
on disease outcome.[1] Nevertheless, these patients cope
with their disease by trusting in the system and in being
'active' in fighting their cancer. It may be hard to wean
such patients off chemotherapy or to stop 'active' treatment as to do so seems, in their eyes, to admit defeat.
Such patients may ask to be put into any trial and see
their role as patients as being fulfilled only so long as
they are participating in active treatment.

'It was not half as bad as I thought it was going to be'

Increasingly, as a result of improved symptom-control
measures and a more holistic approach, patients may
be pleasantly surprised by their tolerance of chemotherapy. Most people have had a previous contact with
someone going through chemotherapy and their
expectations may have been adversely affected by this
experience.

'He has suffered enough'

Other families come through their disease journey
with very ambivalent attitudes towards health care and
oncological treatments. They arrive in the clinic setting
determined that further suffering should be kept
to a minimum. They can be reluctant to consider any
intervention at all, other than the administration of
pain-controlling medications.

'Her hair fell out, then she died'

Many patients and families come with memories and
histories of relatives who have required chemotherapy
in the past. Memories seldom show clearly the distinction between problems caused by the illness itself and
problems caused by side effects. The two merge into a
morass of suffering leaving the patient and the family
convinced that there is only one thing worse than
dying with cancer – and that is dying from cancer with
the side effects of chemotherapy. Doctors and nurses
are not immune to such emotional responses.

'Whatever you say Doctor'

Another group of patients cope with their disease by
investing their trust in 'the doctor' looking after them.
Such an approach runs contrary to non-paternalistic
modern trends but is still present, particularly among
older patients. To present such patients with a meta-
analysis of the benefits of one form of chemotherapy or
another and to ask the patient which one he or she
wants to choose would be inappropriate.

'What about Mexican dog weed?'

Some patients and relatives may come to the clinic
clutching reams of print-outs from the internet about
treatments from clinics around the world. They will
often be very articulate and questioning of every
intervention. Some will have an alternative medicine
approach and be very sceptical of Western medicine.
Honest communication needs to include how health
professionals interpret the clinical research literature
and what they would be prepared to do in terms of
agreeing to provide a treatment that is controversial,
unproven, and unlicensed. Boundaries need to be set
and unrealistic expectations dispelled without remov-
ing hope that a reasonable quality of life can still be
achieved.

'I've had a good life'

A section of patients come into the chemotherapy
clinic without illness at the centre of their lives. Instead
they are focused on their living and their dying with its
important stages and good-byes. Such patients have
accepted the inevitability of their death and have
moved on to preparing for it. They have things that

TABLE 6.2 Classification of anti-cancer agents

Class of agent		Mode of action	Examples in common usage
Cytotoxics	Alkylating agents	Damage DNA by addition of an alkyl group	Cyclophosphamide, ifosfamide, melphalan, busulphan.
	Platinum agents	Damage DNA by addition of platinum adducts	Cisplatin, carboplatin, oxaliplatin
	Antimetabolites	Inhibit production of pyrimidine and purine metabolites	5-Fluorouracil, methotrexate, capecitabine, mercaptopurine, gemcitabine.
	Antitumour antibiotics	Variable	Doxorubicin, epirubicin, mitoxantrone, bleomycin, liposomal anthracyclines
	Vinca alkaloids	Bind to tubulin blocking microtubule and therefore spindle formation at metaphase	Vincristine, vinorelbine, vinblastine
	Taxanes	Promote tubulin polymerization and arrest cells at metaphase	Paclitaxel, docetaxel
	Topoisomerase I inhibitors	Inhibit topoisomerase II leading to DNA damage	Irinotecan, topotecan
Hormonal agents	Selective oestrogen receptor modulators (SERMs)	Partial antagonists of the oestrogen receptor	Tamoxifen
	Aromatase inhibitors	Inhibit extragonadal oestrogen production	Anastrozole, letrozole, exemestane
	Luteinizing hormone releasing hormone (LHRH) agonists	Inhibit gonadal production of oestrogen and testosterone	Leuprolide
	Antiandrogens	Testosterone receptor antagonists	Cyproteron acetate
Immunomodulatory agents	Interferon, interleukin-2		
'Novel' agents	Antibodies	Opsonization, interrupt growth stimulatory pathways	Rituximab, trastuzumab
	Signal transduction inhibitors	Interrupt growth stimulatory pathways	Imatinib, erlotinib, gefitinib, bortezomib
	Vascular targeting agents	Target 'new' vessels associated with tumours	Bevacizumab, thalidomide

they want to do. When it comes to the possibility of chemotherapy for such people their main concern is, 'Will it interfere with what I still have to do?' They are strangely neutral about chemotherapy and it is almost as if they are humouring the professionals by agreeing to it, while they get on with the real business of living.

'I just can't face it'

Some patients have been so worn down by their disease and treatment that the prospect of any more chemotherapy fills them with fear and dread. Sometimes the fears are justified and sometimes they are not.

Sometimes their expression of fear about chemotherapy is a way of verbalizing fears about other matters which should be explored. They face the dilemma of risks and fears whether or not they accept chemotherapy and will need a lot of support in reaching a treatment decision.

Biological therapies

Many anti-cancer agents currently in development have been rationally developed to antagonize elements of the neoplastic process at a cellular level. While most of these agents are still in pre-clinical or early clinical testing a number have already entered routine clinical practice. As a rule these agents are much better tolerated than conventional cytotoxic drugs, with less myelosuppression, alopecia, and emesis. Preclinical testing suggests that many may act as cytostatics rather than cytotoxics and that there may be synergistic interactions with chemotherapy. The challenge in the future will be the rational design of clinical trials to investigate how these agents are best used. There are several types of biological treatment including: monoclonal antibodies, small molecule signaling inhibitors, vaccines, and gene therapy.

Biological therapies can be roughly categorized as:

- Angiogenesis inhibitors
- Cancer growth inhibitors
- Gene therapy
- Vaccines
- Immunotherapy
- Monoclonal antibodies

Angiogenesis inhibitors

Tumours need to produce a network of supporting blood vessels if they are to grow. Angiogenesis inhibitors interfere with the development of blood vessels which in effect starves tumours of oxygen and nutrients. Two such angiogenesis inhibitors are bevacizumab and thalidomide.

Bevacizumab (Avastin®) inhibits angiogenesis by binding to vascular endothelial growth factor (VEGF), the circulating substance that stimulates formation of new blood vessels. This reduces the cancer's supply of oxygen and nutrients, and may also increase vessel permeability allowing better penetration of cytoxics.

Thalidomide is known because of the birth defects caused when it was used to treat sickness in pregnancy in the 1960s. These were caused because thalidomide changes the growth and development of new blood vessels, which is a major attribute in treating malignancy.

Stop and Think

A feature of biological therapies is the trend which they represent of devising treatments which are aimed not just at a specific tumours but at *this* patient's specific tumour cells.

In addition, thalidomide also inhibits tumour necrosis factor. It is most commonly used to treat myeloma.

Cancer growth inhibitors

Advances in the laboratory mean that we now understand many of the processes that drive the growth of cancer cells. These signalling pathways are increasingly being targeted by new drugs. Examples include bortezomib, erlotinib, gefitinib, and imatinib. Some of these molecules bind highly specifically to certain receptors, others affect multiple pathways. Such inhibitors may be used on their own or in combination with chemotherapy.

Bortezomib (Velcade®) inhibits the proteosome, the mechanism by which cells dispose of intracellular peptides. Bortezomib causes a delay in tumour growth and is being used in the treatment of multiple myeloma.

Gefitinib (IRESSA®) and **erlotinib** (Tarceva®). The epidermal growth factor (EGF) receptor is present on the surface of many normal cells but overexpressed or mutated in a range of epithelial cancers to the EGF receptor tyrosine kinase inside the cell and prevent the receptor from being activated. This switches off important signalling pathways that drive processes fundamental to the cancer cell (e.g. proliferation). Both erlotinib and gefitinib cause tumour shrinkage in a limited proportion of patients with non-small cell lung cancer and stabilise disease in many more. Erlotinib in particular is being used increasingly in these patients, its main side effect being an acne-like skin rash.

Imatinib (Glivec®) is a signal transduction inhibitor inhibiting the Bcr-abl receptor tyrosine kinase characteristic of chronic myeloid leukaemia (CML) and c kit receptor tyrosine kinase associated with gastrointestinal stromal tumours (GIST). Imatinib has dramatically changed the treatment of CML and GIST. Other tyrosine kinase inhibitors entering the clinic include sorafinib (renal cancer) and sunitinib (for relapsed renal cancers and GIST). Both are active against multiple kinases.

Gene therapy

Gene therapy involves inserting DNA into cells so that the cells can produce new proteins to help fight disease. Single genes can be taken from human cells and cloned in the laboratory. These cloned genes can be altered to make them work differently. Such altered genes can be put back into cells by inserting the gene using vectors such as liposomes or attenuated viruses. Gene therapy is still experimental with studies focusing on the safety aspects of such treatment.

Immunotherapy

Interferon (interferon alpha; Introna®, Roferon-A®)

There are three main types of interferon: alpha, beta, and gamma. Interferon is used in the treatment of cancer of the kidney, malignant melanoma, multiple myeloma, carcinoid tumours, and some types of lymphoma and leukaemia. It is given to stimulate the body's own immune system. Interferon has a wide range of biological effects. It may do one or more of the following:

♦ Slow down or stop cancer cells dividing

♦ Reduce the ability of cancer cells to protect themselves from the immune system

♦ Strengthen the body's immune system

Aldesleukin (Proleukin®) used to be known as interleukin-2 or IL-2 and is a cytokine produced by T lymphocytes to stimulate the body's own defence mechanism. It has been used in the treatment of renal carcinoma and malignant melanoma.

Vaccines

The aim of cancer vaccines is to stimulate the immune system to be able to recognize cancer cells as abnormal and destroy them. Cancer vaccines are made from the person's own cancer cells or from cells that are grown in a laboratory and are then attenuated by heat or radiation. Both specific cell antigens as well as occasionally whole cells are used to make a vaccine.

Trials are mainly being carried out on patients who have advanced cancers and a wide range of malignancies have been studied. To date, such vaccines have not proved effective. An alternative approach that may be more effective is to vaccinate against the cause of cancer in the rare cases where a viral cause is known (e.g. human papillomavirus in cervical cancer).

Monoclonal antibodies

Cancer cells often over-express specific cell surface receptor proteins that straddle the cell membrane. The extracellular portion binds to circulating ligands and this activates the intracellular tyrosine kinase portion that stimulates signalling pathways inside the cancer cell. A monoclonal antibody recognizes the receptor on the outer surface of cancer cells and 'locks' on to it. This can:

♦ Trigger the body's immune system to attack the cancer cells and cause the cells to destroy themselves

♦ Stop the receptor from connecting with a different protein that helps the cell to grow, which may stop the cells from growing and dividing, or prevent the cancer cells from developing a new blood supply

Trastuzumab (Herceptin®) attaches itself to the Her-2 protein, thereby inhibiting cell growth. Trastuzumab also stimulates the body's own immune responses to cancer cells, and has a clear synergistic effect along with paclitaxel (Taxol®) or docetaxel (Taxotere®) chemotherapy. However, 20% of breast cancers over-express the Her-2 receptor, making them suitable for treatment with Herceptin®. It is, therefore, important that all breast cancers be tested for Her-2 positivity in order to identify those women who may benefit from trastuzumab in either the adjunctive or metastatic setting. Trastuzumab is generally well tolerated and adds little to the toxicity of chemotherapy when given with cytotoxics. The exception is that trastuzumab does carry a significant risk of cardiac toxicity when given with an anthracycline. A major issue for prescribing trastuzumab is the cost of £25,000 per year. Another issue has been the UK post code lottery affecting its availability in the adjuvant setting.

Rituximab (MabThera®) is used to treat several types of non-Hodgkin's lymphoma. It can be given on its own to people who cannot have chemotherapy because of the potential side effects, or to those whose lymphoma has come back after chemotherapy.[3] It can also be given in combination with chemotherapy as the first treatment for people who have high-grade lymphoma that is at an advanced stage when first diagnosed. Rituximab locks on to a protein called CD20 which is found on the surface of B-cell lymphocytes. CD20 is also present on the surface of most abnormal B-cell lymphocytes which occur in most types of non-Hodgkin's lymphoma.

Thus rituximab attacks both malignant and normal B-cell lymphocytes. However, the body quickly replaces any normal white blood cells which are damaged.

Bevacizumab (Avastin®) does not bind to a cell surface receptor. Rather, it inhibits angiogenesis by binding to circulating VEGF. This reduces the stimulus for new vessel formation and may 'starve' the tumour. It also affects the permeability of abnormal tumour vasculature, reducing interstitial pressure and potentially allowing cytotoxics to enter the tumour more effectively. Bevacizumab increases the efficacy of chemotherapy in patients with a range of cancers, for example, bowel, breast, and lung cancers.

Cetuximab (Erbitux®) attaches itself to the extracellular portion of the EGF receptor (in contrast to gefitinib or erlotinib, which act on its intracellular tyrosine kinase) preventing the receptor from being activated. This stops the cells from dividing. Cetuximab may also make the cancer cells more sensitive to chemotherapy. It is also used to treat advanced colorectal cancer in patients who have demonstrable EGF receptor. Cetuximab is given in combination with the chemotherapy drug irinotecan. It is also being used in trials to treat other types of cancer, including non-small cell lung cancer and cancer of the head and neck. Cetuximab may be used on its own or with radiotherapy.[4]

Test Yourself

How would you answer a young mother with early breast cancer who asks to be given Herceptin® (trastuzumab) as she has heard that it will really improve her chances of long-term survival?

TABLE 6.3 Commonly used anti-cancer drugs (new drugs being introduced regularly)

Drug	Administration	Excretion	Side effects	Common indications[a]
Bleomycin *Cytotoxic antibiotic*	IV	Renal	'Flu symptoms' Hyperpigmentation Allergic reactions Pulmonary fibrosis (common with doses > 300 mg)	Germ cell tumours Lymphoma
Busulphan *Alkylating agent*	PO	Renal	Myelosuppression Hyperpigmentation Pulmonary interstitial fibrosis Hepato-venous occlusion	Leukaemia
Carboplatin	IV	Renal	Myelosuppression especially thrombocytopenia. Emesis	Ovarian cancer Lung
Capecitabine *Anti-metabolite*	PO	Renal	Hand–foot syndrome Stomatitis Diarrhoea	Colorectal cancer Breast cancer
Cisplatin	IV	Renal	Emesis Renal failure Peripheral neuropathy Ototoxicity Allergic reactions	Germ cell tumours Lung cancer Ovary
Cyclophosphamide *Alkylating agent*	PO	Hepatic and renal	Myelosuppression Alopecia Emesis Haemorrhagic cystitis	Breast cancer Lymphoma
Cytarabine *Anti-metabolite*	IV, IT, SC	Hepatic and renal	Myelosuppression Diarrhoea Stomatitis	Leukaemia
Dactinomycin *Cytotoxic antibiotic*	IV	Hepatic and renal	Myelosuppression Mucositis Diarrhoea Alopecia	Choriocarcinoma Ewing's sarcoma Wilms' tumour Paediatric tumours
Docetaxel *Taxane*	IV	Hepatic	Myelosuppression Fluid retention Alopecia Peripheral neuropathy	Breast cancer

TABLE 6.3 Commonly used anti-cancer drugs (new drugs being introduced regularly) – *continued*

Drug	Administration	Excretion	Side effects	Common indications[a]
Doxorubicin	IV and intravesical	Hepatic	Emesis	Breast cancer
			Myelosuppression	Sarcoma
			Mucositis	
			Alopecia	
Cytotoxic antibiotic			Cardiomyopathy (risk related to total cumulative dose)	
Epirubicin *Cytotoxic antibiotic*	IV	Hepatic	Similar to doxorubicin but less cardiotoxic	Breast cancer
Etoposide	IV, PO	Renal	Myelosuppression	Lung cancer
			Emesis	Germ cell tumour
Topoisomerase II inhibitor			Alopecia	
			Secondary leukaemia	
Fluorouracil	IV, topical cream	Liver and renal	Mucositis	Colorectal cancer
			Diarrhoea	Breast cancer
			Hand–foot syndrome	etc.
			Myelosuppression	
			Gastrointestinal upsets	
			Cerebellar ataxia (rare)	
Anti-metabolite			Gritty eyes and blurred vision	
Gemcitabine	IV	Renal	Myelosuppression	Pancreatic cancer
			'Flu-like' symptoms	Bladder cancer
			Fatigue	Lung cancer
Anti-metabolite			Pneumonitis	
Ifosfamide	IV	Hepatic and renal	Alopecia	Sarcomas
			Emesis	Lung
			Haemorrhagic cystitis	
Alkylating agent			Encephalopathy	
Irinotecan	IV	Hepatic and renal	Cholinergic syndrome (associated with infusion)	Colorectal cancer
			Delayed diarrhoea	
			Nausea and vomiting	
			Myelosuppression	
Topoisomerase inhibitor			Alopecia	
Liposomal anthracycline	IV	Hepatic	Hand–foot syndrome	Ovarian cancer
			Stomatitis	Breast cancer
				Kaposi's sarcoma

TABLE 6.3 Commonly used anti-cancer drugs (new drugs being introduced regularly) – *continued*

Drug	Administration	Excretion	Side effects	Common indications[a]
Mercaptopurine *Anti-metabolite*	PO	Peripheral tissues	Myelosuppression Hepatic dysfunction Stomatitis	Leukaemia
Methotrexate Folic acid analogue *Anti-metabolite*	PO, IV, IM, IT	Renal	Myelosuppression Mucositis Skin pigmentation Nephrotoxicity	Osteosarcoma Breast cancer Leukaemia Lymphoma
Mitomycin C *Cytotoxic antibiotic*	IV or intravesical	Hepatic metabolism	Myelosuppression Lung fibrosis Nephrotoxicity Stomatitis Diarrhoea Haemolytic uraemic syndrome	Anal Bladder
Mitoxantrone *Cytotoxic antibiotic*	IV	Bile > urine	Myelosuppression Emesis Alopecia Mucositis Cardiotoxicity	Lymphoma Leukaemia
Oxaliplatin *DNA binder*	IV	Renal	Peripheral neuropathy Myelosuppression Nausea and vomiting Laryngeal spasm	Colorectal cancer
Paclitaxel	IV	Hepatic	Myelosuppression Alopecia Hypersensitivity reactions Peripheral neuropathy	Ovarian cancer Lung cancer Breast cancer
Pemetrexed IV	IV	Renal	Myelosuppression Rash Stomatitis Drowsiness	Mesothelioma (in combination with platinum)
Temozolamide *Alkylating agent*	PO		Emesis Myelosuppression	Astrocytomas Melanoma
Thioguanine *Anti-metabolite*	PO	Renal	Myelosuppression Mucositis Diarrhoea Hepatic dysfunction	Leukaemia

TABLE 6.3 Commonly used anti-cancer drugs (new drugs being introduced regularly) – *continued*

Drug	Administration	Excretion	Side effects	Common indications[a]
Thiotepa *Alkylating agent*	IV	Excreted more in urine than bile	Myelosuppression	Leukaemia
Topotecan *Topoisomerase inhibitor*	IV	Liver metabolism Urine excretion	Myelosuppression Emesis Alopecia Diarrhoea	Ovarian cancer
Vinblastine *Mitotic spindle inhibitor*	IV	Hepatic	Myelosuppression Constipation Stomatitis Rare: hair loss or peripheral neurotoxicity	Lymphoma Germ cell tumours
Vincristine *Mitotic spindle inhibitor*	IV	Hepatic	Peripheral neuropathy Autonomic neuropathy	Leukaemia Lymphoma
Vindesine *Mitotic spindle inhibitor*	IV	Hepatic	Myelosuppression Mild neurotoxicity Autonomic neuropathy	Leukaemia
Vinorelbine *Mitotic spindle inhibitor*	IV	Hepatic	Myelosuppression Phlebitis Peripheral neuropathy	Breast cancer Non-small cell lung cancer

IV, intravenous; PO, per os (by mouth); IT, intrathecal; SC, subcutaneous; IM, intramuscular
[a]Often used for tumours other than those officially licensed.

TABLE 6.4 Hormone and anti-hormone drugs

Drug	Administration	Side effects	Comments
Selective oestrogen receptor modulators	PO	Menopausal symptoms Thromboembolic event Endometrial hyperplasia and cancer	Used first-line in adjuvant treatment of ER/PR +ve breast cancer
Tamoxifen			
Fulvestrant (Pure oestrogen receptor, antagonist)	IM	Menopausal symptoms	Post menopausal ER/PR +ve breast cancer
Anti-androgens	PO	Hepatotoxicity	Used in prostate cancer, sometimes in combination with GNRH analogues
Bicalutamide		Gynaecomastia	
Cyproterone acetate			
Flutamide			
Aromatase inhibitors		Menopausal symptoms Increased fractures	Used in post-menopausal breast cancer
Anastrozole	PO		
Letrozole	PO		
Exemestane	PO		
Formestane	IM		
GNRH analogues		Gynaecomastia, impotence, nausea, fluid retention	Prostate cancer Breast cancer
Buserelin	SC and intranasal	Menopausal symptoms	
Goserelin	Implant		
Leuprorelin	IM		
Triptorelin	IM		

PO, per os; SC, subcutaneous; IM, intramuscular; GNRH, gonadotrophin-releasing hormone.

TABLE 6.5 Emetic risk of common chemotherapy drugs

Cytotoxic agents	Risk
Cisplatin*	
Cyclophosphamide > 1,000 mg/m²*	High
Ifosfamide*	
Melphalan*	
Actinomycin	
Amsacrine	
Busulphan	
Carboplatin*	
Chlorambucil	
Cladribine	
Cyclophosphamide < 1,000 mg/m²	
Cytarabine > 150 mg/m²	
Dacarbazine	Moderate
Daunorubicin	
Daunorubicin liposomal	
Doxorubicin	
Epirubicin	
Lomustine	
Methotrexate > 1 g/m²	
Mitozantrone	
Procarbazine	
Bleomycin	
Capecitabine	
Cyclophosphamide < 300 mg/m²	
Cytarabine < 150 mg/m²	
Etoposide	
5-Fluorouracil	
Fludarabine	
Mercaptopurine	Low
Methotrexate < 1 g/m²	
Thioguanine	
Thiotepa	
Vinblastine	
Vincristine	

* Delayed emesis risk

Chapter summary

- Tumours which divide rapidly with short doubling times usually respond best to chemotherapy
- Chemotherapy drugs influence different phases of the cell cycle
- The probability of cure with chemotherapy is inversely proportional to the tumour burden
- The ability of cells to either repair or tolerate the damage inflicted by chemotherapy may lead to chemoresistance
- Chemotherapy may be given in the following settings:
  - Neo-adjuvant (before local treatment)
  - Adjuvant (after local treatment)
  - Metastatic (for widespread disease)
- The decision to use chemotherapy is often a complex matter and a number of factors must be taken into consideration
- Biological therapies/immunotherapy are increasingly being used to target treatment to specific tumour types
- Modes of action of these treatments include:
  - Angiogenesis inhibition
  - Cancer growth inhibitors
  - Gene therapy
  - Vaccines
  - Immunotherapy
  - Monoclonal antibody treatments

References

1. Petticrew M, *et al*. Influence of psychological coping on survival and recurrence in people with cancer: systematic review. *BMJ* 2002, **325**, 1066.
2. Full guidance on trastuzumab for advanced breast cancer. National Institute for Clinical Excellence (NICE), March 2002.
3. Full guidance on rituximab for aggressive non-Hodgkin's lymphoma. National Institute for Clinical Excellence (NICE), September 2003. Full guidance on rituximab for follicular non-Hodgkin's lymphoma. National Institute for Clinical Excellence (NICE), March 2002.
4. Cunningham D, *et al*. Cetuximab monotherapy and cetuximab plus irinotecan in irinotecan-refractory metastatic colorectal cancer. *New England Journal of Medicine* 2004, **351**, 337–45.

Radiotherapy

Chapter contents

Key Facts

Clinical oncologists specialize in the use of radiotherapy and also use chemotherapy.

Medical oncologists specialize in the use of chemotherapy and do not use radiotherapy.

Introduction

Radiotherapy as a therapeutic modality developed shortly after the discovery of X-rays at the end of the nineteenth century. Clinical and technological advances subsequently have made it one of the most successful modalities in the treatment of patients with cancer, both in curative and palliative settings.

'Radiotherapy is used for about half of the 250,000 patients who develop cancer in the UK each year. It has a curative role in two-thirds, and a palliative role in the remainder.'

Professor Alan Horwich, Royal Marsden

Mechanism of action

Radiotherapy is the therapeutic use of ionizing radiation to damage cancerous cells. The critical cellular target is, in common with chemotherapy, nuclear DNA. Double-stranded breaks in the DNA molecule appear to be the lesion responsible for cell death. Cell death takes place during subsequent mitotic cell division, hence the term mitotic cell death. Much less commonly, certain tissue types, such as lymphocytes and parotid acinar cells, undergo cell death without attempting mitosis, a process known as interphase cell death. Not all double-stranded DNA breaks, however, result in cell death. Indeed, most are repaired by the cell's DNA repair enzyme apparatus. The success or otherwise of these repair processes determines the fate of the cell.

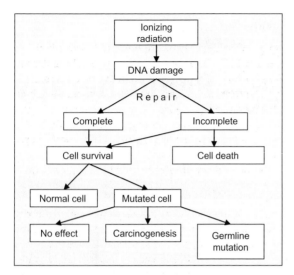

Fig. 7.1 Ionizing radiation effects.

> **Key Fact**
>
> Radiation is relatively less effective in an environment that is poorly oxygenated.

Response of normal tissues to radiation

Different normal tissues vary in their response to radiation. Homeostatic mechanisms control cell populations by balancing cell death with new cell growth through the proliferation of progenitor cells derived from stem cells. If a proportion of these stem cells are destroyed by radiation, the rate of renewal of normal cells will be reduced. The time of appearance of this tissue damage is determined by the lifespan of the mature cells within that tissue. For certain tissues, such as skin and mucosa, this lifespan is short because cells are quickly lost by desquamation; hence, tissue damage is manifest during the radiation course. For other tissues, cell turnover is much slower and radiation damage may only become apparent many months or years after radiation exposure. This gives rise to the distinction between the acute and late effects of irradiation.

Acute effects of radiation

These are the normal tissue reactions during or within 90 days of starting a course of radiotherapy. The mucosa and haemopoietic system, i.e. tissues with a fast normal cellular turnover, display effects of irradiation earliest. For example, patients undergoing radiotherapy to the head and neck may develop severe oral mucositis, whereas those receiving radiotherapy to significant volumes of bone marrow may develop bone marrow suppression.

Acute reactions are usually observed during the course of conventionally fractionated radiotherapy (1.8–2 Gy per fraction five times a week).

Late effects of radiation

These occur predominantly in slowly proliferating tissues (lung, kidney, heart, liver, and central nervous system). By definition, late reactions occur more than 90 days after commencing a course of radiation.

Consequential late effects

Some of the tissues which develop their effects early can also demonstrate late effects such as fibrosis or telangiectasia in the skin. This reflects the differing populations of cells (fibroblasts, endothelium etc.) that exist within a single organ.

Radiotherapy may be administered in differing clinical situations and with varying intents:

- **Radical** – curative intent
- **Adjuvant** – post-operative
- **Palliative** – symptom control

Radical radiotherapy

Radiotherapy may be administered with the intent of cure either as the preferred primary therapy (e.g. early stage Hodgkin's disease), or as an alternative to surgery.

In the latter situation it has the advantage of preserving normal anatomy, e.g. anal canal cancer, prostatic cancer, laryngeal cancer, and bladder cancer. Additionally, acute morbidity is often less severe. However, as no surgical specimen is obtained, there can be no pathological data to permit accurate staging.

TABLE 7.1	Three types of radiation therapy
Type	**Examples**
External beam radiotherapy (delivered by radiotherapy machines)	Breast and pelvic tumours
Brachytherapy (sealed-source radiation)	Cervical, head and neck tumours
Unsealed source or radioisotope therapy (given by mouth, intravenously or into tissue spaces)	Iodine[131] – thyroid tumours Strontium[89] – bone metastases

Stop and Think

Once an area of tissue has received the maximum tolerable dosage of radiotherapy it cannot usually be irradiated again as further irradiation may cause serious damage to normal tissues within the field of irradiation.

Stage must therefore be assessed by clinical or radiological methods. Late effects of radiation, such as fibrosis, may also make subsequent assessment of the tumour site for local recurrence difficult, clinically, radiologically, and pathologically.

Radical radiation is reserved for tumours that can be encompassed within a reasonable radiation treatment volume, i.e. localized, as opposed to widely metastatic disease; this presupposes accurate staging investigations.

Treatment is often complex with effort given to immobilization of the patient/tumour and the use of complicated beam arrangements to obtain a uniform dose distribution confined to the tumour rather than normal surrounding structures. A high dose of radiation is necessary for all but the most radiosensitive of tumours; treatment is delivered in small daily fractions, typically over up to 7 weeks to reduce late adverse effects.

Radical radiotherapy can be used in various tumours.

Head and neck cancer

Many squamous cell tumours of the head and neck can be cured by radical radiotherapy (often combined with synchronous chemotherapy); for example, early stage cancers of the larynx are frequently cured with preservation of good quality phonation, which is lost with surgery.

Anal canal cancer

A radical approach using concurrent chemo-radiotherapy is effective for epidermoid anal canal cancer. Between 60 and 70% of patients retain a functioning anal sphincter after treatment. The alternative is primary abdominoperineal excision of the rectum and anal canal, which results in a permanent colostomy.

Lung cancer

Radical radiotherapy is employed in the management of non-small cell lung cancer when patients are not deemed sufficiently fit to undergo radical surgery.

Adjuvant radiotherapy

Adjuvant radiotherapy is administered as an adjunct to potentially curative surgery. The principle underpinning such treatment is the possibility that microscopic residual disease, either within the tumour bed, lymphatic channels, or regional lymph nodes, remains after surgery. Adjuvant radiotherapy aims to eradicate this microscopic disease, reducing the rate of local relapse and improving overall survival.

Examples of adjuvant radiotherapy are given below.

Breast cancer

This is perhaps the best and certainly most commonly used example of adjuvant radiation. Up to 50% of the workload of many UK radiotherapy centres is devoted to adjuvant breast irradiation. Local relapse rates following partial mastectomy may reach 30%. Postoperative breast irradiation can reduce this figure by three- to four-fold. Local control rates then conform to those achieved after mastectomy but with a better cosmetic outcome.

Head and neck cancer

Surgery for squamous tumours of the head and neck is complex. The close proximity of tumours to important structures means that surgical margins may often be inadequate because a compromise must be made between retaining acceptable function and obtaining a good cosmetic outcome. Adjuvant irradiation is used if the margins are unsatisfactory or where radical neck surgery demonstrates multiple involved lymph nodes.

Classically, adjuvant radiotherapy is administered after surgery. However, in some situations, although surgery remains the mainstay of treatment, radiotherapy may be delivered as a prelude to a surgical procedure.

True neo-adjuvant radiation is administered to shrink or 'downstage' the tumour, thus facilitating subsequent surgery. In this situation, time must elapse between irradiation and surgery to allow tumour reduction. An illustration of this approach is preoperative rectal radiotherapy for tethered or fixed rectal adenocarcinoma. Treatment is delivered over 4–5 weeks after which there is a gap of about 6 weeks during which tumour shrinkage occurs. Surgery is then often possible when it would not have been before radiotherapy.

Short-course preoperative rectal radiotherapy, by contrast, is delivered over the week immediately prior to surgery with the goal of 'sterilizing' the tumour before surgical manipulation. No time is allowed for tumour shrinkage. Trials have, however, confirmed a significant improvement in local control and overall survival with this approach, although there are concerns about increased risk of late effects with this short treatment.

Adjuvant radiation treatment courses typically extend over 4–7 weeks. The general principles applied to radical radiotherapy also hold for the adjuvant setting as treatment intent is curative, i.e. immobilization, careful avoidance of critical organs at risk, and low dose per fraction. Total doses tend to be slightly lower since the target is microscopic residual disease. It must, however, be remembered that following surgery, the vascular supply to tissues is disrupted, resulting in areas of tissue hypoxia which may be more resistant to radiation effects.

Palliative radiotherapy

When radiotherapy is administered in the palliative setting, the focus of interest is the control of distressing symptoms. The disease is, by definition, incurable. These factors impact upon treatment in a variety of ways:

- Only symptomatic sites of disease are targeted
- Fractionation regimens are kept short
- Moderate doses of radiation are employed
- Palliative benefit must outweigh treatment-related toxicity

Palliative radiotherapy may produce prolongation of survival but this is not its primary aim, rather it is the quality of that survival that is the goal. Palliative radiotherapy often produces significant symptomatic gain. In addition, anticipating problems that are likely to cause symptoms and treating before the patient becomes symptomatic may be beneficial.

There are several clinical scenarios in which palliative radiotherapy commonly proves useful:

Pain

Bone metastases and pain due to nerve compression or soft tissue infiltration will usually respond to radiation treatment given in large single fractions of radiotherapy as well as to the more prolonged treatment schedules.

The former are more patient friendly and may be repeated if necessary. If pain is diffuse, affecting many sites within the skeleton, wide-field – hemibody – irradiation often produces relief. An alternative is radioisotope therapy with strontium[89] or samarium[153] both of which are administered systemically.

Osteolytic tumour deposits in weight-bearing bones are at risk of fracture and are best fixed prophylactically by orthopaedic intervention. This is often followed by post-operative irradiation although good evidence of benefit is lacking. In some specific situations radiation is given without prophylactic surgical intervention.

Haemorrhage

Haemoptysis, haematuria, haematemesis, and rectal bleeding can be reduced by radiation. A hypofractionated treatment course often produces prompt sustained benefit (in at least 70% of patients with lung cancer). Hypofractionation involves fewer fractions of radiotherapy but bigger doses per fraction.

Obstruction

Any hollow viscus may undergo obstruction caused by cancer. Several organs are commonly involved in this way:

- Superior vena cava
- Upper airways, i.e. trachea, bronchus
- Oesophagus

Prompt, if not immediate, relief is frequently afforded by stent insertion under the care of the interventional radiologists for superior vena canal or oesophageal obstruction. There is a role for palliative radiotherapy in some patients who are unsuitable for such procedures or in the case of stent overgrowth by tumour.

Radiotherapy is most often used for bronchial obstruction resulting from lung cancer; laser resection or stent insertion are less commonly employed alternatives. Endoluminal radiotherapy may be used to control tumour with a single treatment.

Radiotherapy probably remains the treatment modality of choice for obstruction of the superior vena cava caused by radio-sensitive tumours, for example, small cell lung cancer.

Neurological symptoms

- Spinal cord compression
- Brain metastases
- Cranial or peripheral nerve compression
- Choroidal or orbital metastases

Radiotherapy is the most common means of treating spinal cord compression. There are a number of important indications for surgical as opposed to radiotherapeutic intervention (e.g. uncertain pathology, unstable spine).

Radiotherapy often improves pain associated with spinal compression, but neurological recovery is less

Key Fact

Radiotherapy is not used to relieve bowel obstruction secondary to gastrointestinal or ovarian malignancy because such obstruction often involves multiple sites and normal adjacent tissues are very easily damaged, making the situation worse through oedema and fibrosis. In such circumstances stents may be employed.

predictable and mainly depends on the degree of weakness prior to therapy and the particular histological tumour type. A patient who comes to the hospital incontinent or in a wheel chair is unlikely to leave hospital neurologically intact so early diagnosis and treatment are vital.

Brain metastases are increasing in incidence as oncological management improves and patients survive long enough to relapse with metastases in the brain. Steroids can produce significant symptomatic benefit if the effects are the result of oedema or compression rather than tissue destruction. However, their beneficial effects tend to be short-lived. Prolongation of symptom control and a small gain in survival (1–2 months) can be obtained with cranial irradiation, usually at the cost of alopecia and lethargy. Those patients with good pre-treatment neurological function and radio-sensitive tumours stand to gain most.

Cranial or peripheral nerve compression most often occurs with breast or prostate neoplasms. Pain is often improved but nerve palsies seldom show significant recovery.

Fungating tumours

Locally advanced breast tumours, skin tumours, metastatic skin or lymph node deposits, can all lead the disease to fungate or erupt through the skin. If surgery is not possible or felt to be inappropriate, radiotherapy can reduce the tumour mass, serous ooze or haemorrhage, and may promote healing.

Managing side effects of radiotherapy

Side effects of radiotherapy are most obviously localized rather than systemic. However, chronic toxicity can be a more hidden problem particularly following high doses of curative and adjuvant radiotherapy.

Skin

General advice

- Skin reactions tend to be worse in the skin folds, i.e. inframammary fold, axilla, groin, and perineum

- Deodorants should be avoided within the treatment area
- Avoid aftershave lotions or astringent cosmetics
- Mild soaps are permitted, and washing should be gentle (no vigorous rubbing) and the area patted dry
- Care must be taken not to remove skin markings delineating the treatment fields

Mild reactions

- Skin pink or slightly red
- Apply aqueous cream frequently

Moderate reactions

- Skin red, dry, and scaly; some pruritus/tingling
- Apply aqueous cream frequently
- If itch is problematic, 1% hydrocortisone cream q.d.s. is useful

Severe reactions

- Skin inflamed/patchy areas of moist desquamation
- Epidermis may blister and slough exposing the dermis leading to pain and serous ooze with increased risk of infection
- Hydrogel or alginate dressing to moist areas; Diprobase® cream to intact epidermis
- Swab if evidence of infection

Mouth and throat care

This is particularly important for patients receiving radiotherapy to the head and neck.

General advice

- The patient needs a dental assessment and any dental treatment should be carried out before radiotherapy begins
- A good fluid and nutritional intake is very important and nutritional support by nasogastric tube
- Percutaneous endoscopic gastrostomy or radiologically introduced gastrostomy is indicated if > 10% weight loss occurs
- Cessation of smoking should be strongly encouraged
- Alcohol and spicy foods should be avoided
- The voice should be rested as the radiotherapy reaction becomes established

Treatment of mucositis

- Normal saline or bicarbonate mouth washes often help

- Antiseptic mouth washes, e.g. chlorhexidine, keep the mouth clean but can cause pain because of their alcohol content

- Oropharyngeal infection with *Candida* should be actively sought and treated

- Local analgesics include:
  - Aspirin (which may be gargled)
  - Paracetamol (which may be gargled)
  - Benzydamine (Difflam®)
  - Local anaesthetics (Xylocaine®)
  - Topical steroids (Adcortyl in Orobase®, Corlan pellets®)
  - Coating agents (sucralfate, Gelclair®)

Dysphagia

Thoracic radiotherapy can lead to oesophagitis which needs explanation and symptomatic treatment.

Smoking should be strongly discouraged; spirits and spicy food should be avoided.

An antacid, e.g. Gaviscon®, soluble paracetamol or aspirin may all help. A non-steroidal anti-inflammatory drug either orally or by suppository may be used. The oesophagus can be coated with some effect by sucralfate.

Nausea and vomiting

Radiotherapy to the abdomen often causes nausea as a result of serotonin release. All patients should be considered for prophylactic anti-emetic therapy, e.g. ondansetron.

Diarrhoea

This frequently accompanies radiotherapy to the abdomen or pelvis.

Dietary modification, i.e. reduction in dietary roughage, may sometimes relieve the diarrhoea.

Anti-diarrhoeal drugs (e.g. loperamide) should be provided for all patients with clear instructions of when and how they should be taken.

Proctitis often accompanies rectal or prostatic irradiation and should be treated with rectal steroids either by suppository or enema.

Pneumonitis

Acute radiotherapy-induced pneumonitis can develop 1–3 months after treatment and is associated with a fever, dry cough, and breathlessness. The main differential diagnosis is pneumonia. The diagnosis can be confirmed by a chest X-ray, which shows lung infiltration confined within the treatment volume. Treatment is with a reducing course of steroids, i.e. a starting dose of prednisolone 40 mg.

Cerebral oedema

This can occur during or after cranial irradiation, particularly if no surgical decompression of the brain tumour or metastasis has been undertaken. Oedema usually responds to an increase in the dose of oral steroids, the dose being reduced following the completion of radiotherapy.

Somnolence syndrome

This occurs within a few weeks of completion of brain irradiation and may manifest itself with nausea, vomiting, anorexia, dysarthria, ataxia, and profound lethargy. Recovery may occur spontaneously.

New developments

Radiotherapy has advanced markedly since the early days of the twentieth century. Progress is still being made to improve the quality and effectiveness of treatment for patients.

There are a number of areas of development:

Defining tumour volume

Improvements in imaging have enabled tumours to be targeted more accurately. This reduces the risk of missing the tumour, and also allows the treatment volume to encompass the tumour more closely. The dose of radiation can therefore be higher (giving improved tumour control) without risking additional toxicity to normal tissues.

Imaging

Refinements in computerized tomography (CT) scanning technology have led to the advent of the multi-slice CT scanner that provides multiple high-quality images rapidly, from which tumour volumes may be defined in three dimensions.

Images can now be fused from different imaging modalities, e.g. magnetic resonance imaging/CT image fusion. The development of co-registered CT/positron emission tomography (PET) scanning combines functional data (from PET scanning) and high-quality spatial information (from CT scanning), providing opportunity for optimal target volume definition.

Conformal therapy

Imaging improvements provide the ability to identify the tumour target more accurately. This reduces the risk of missing the tumour, but it also provides the opportunity of conforming the treatment more closely to the tumour volume and thereby lessening damage to surrounding normal tissues. Taken further, conformal therapy may permit dose escalation with resulting improved tumour control rates, but without increased toxicity. Multileaf collimators within the treatment unit can automatically shape the treatment field, conforming it to the desired target shape.

Intensity modulated radiotherapy (IMRT)

With IMRT the intensity of the treatment beams are modified in such a way that almost any three-dimensional volume may be generated. Even concave volumes may be created and so targets which envelop the spinal cord, e.g. thyroid, can be treated much more satisfactorily than with conventional techniques.

Fractionation/combined modality treatment

Advances in the understanding of the principles of fractionation have led to improved treatment outcomes for patients, e.g. CHART (continuous hyperfractionated accelerated radiotherapy) in non-small cell lung cancer. Further research with hypo/hyper-fractionation and acceleration is ongoing in other tumour types.

The integration of chemotherapy with radiation treatment has provided benefit in a number of tumour sites, e.g. cervical cancer. Research seeks to refine this further and also to incorporate the newer molecular agents into radiation therapy.

Individualization of therapy

Two patients with ostensibly similar tumours receiving identical treatments may respond differently, one being cured and the other dying from cancer in a short time. There are clearly factors inherent within tumours which predict for response to radiotherapy. If such variables could be identified before a treatment course commences, the chance of response would be defined, which would help clinicians in deciding whether or not radiotherapy would be a good treatment option. Furthermore, it might be possible, knowing the particular tumour characteristics, to adapt the treatment course accordingly, perhaps by modifying the dose

prescribed, or altering the fractionation schedule so that the prospect of cure could be enhanced. Predictive assays are being developed to realize this possibility. New microchip technology may help elucidate the genes behind the differing responses to therapy, and more importantly, offer patients the possibility of treatment tailored to their individual needs.

Chapter summary

- Radiotherapy is the therapeutic use of ionizing radiation to damage cancerous cells
- Different types of normal tissue respond differently to radiation
- Tissues with a fast normal cellular turnover display the effects of irradiation earliest
- Late effects of radiation occur predominantly in slowly proliferating tissues (lung, kidney, heart, liver, and central nervous system)
- Re-treating areas that have already received a maximal radiation dose should be avoided
- There are three main types of radiation therapy:
  - External beam radiotherapy (delivered by radiotherapy machines)
  - Brachytherapy (solid radiation sources inserted directly into tumours)
  - Unsealed source or radioisotope therapy (given by mouth, intravenously, or into tissue spaces)
- During the process of treatment planning questions such as 'where to treat?', 'what to treat?', 'what not to treat?', 'how to treat?' and 'how much to treat?' are addressed
- Fractionation is used to permit repair of normal tissue radiation damage
- Three constituents make up a radiotherapy prescription:
  - Total dose
  - Number of fractions (fraction size)
  - Overall treatment time
- Unsealed source therapy involves administering radioactive substances directly into the patient either in the form of liquids for ingestion or solutions for intravenous administration

Chapter summary—*cont'd.*

- Radical radiotherapy may be administered with the intent of cure either as the preferred primary therapy (e.g. laryngeal cancer), or as an alternative to surgery
- Adjuvant radiotherapy is administered as an adjunct to potentially curative surgery
- Neo-adjuvant radiation is administered to shrink or downstage the tumour, facilitating subsequent surgery
- When radiotherapy is administered in the palliative setting the focus of interest is the control of distressing symptoms

Patients with lung cancer

Incidence and mortality

In 2001 22,700 men and 14,700 women were diagnosed with lung cancer in the UK.[1]

In 2003 19,800 men and 13, 600 women died from lung cancer in the UK.[2]

Background

♦ Most common cancer in men and women in UK and USA

♦ 80% are the result of smoking

♦ Small cell lung cancers (SCLC) comprise 25%

♦ Non-small cell lung cancers (NSCLC) comprise the remaining 75%

• Squamous cell carcinoma 30%

• Adenocarcinoma (including bronchioalveolar carcinoma) 35%

• Large cell anaplastic carcinoma 10%

Natural history

♦ The pattern of growth is related to cell histology

• Adenocarcinomas grow slowly

• Small cell carcinoma metastasizes early with 80–90% having spread beyond the thorax at the time of diagnosis

♦ Lung cancer spreads circumferentially and longitudinally along the bronchus and may lead to bronchial occlusion and lobar collapse with associated pneumonia or empyema

♦ Mediastinal structures, oesophagus, pericardium, and great vessels can become involved

- Common sites of metastases include:
  - Liver
  - Brain
  - Bone
  - There is an unusual and unexplained propensity for adrenal gland involvement
  - Lung
  - Skin

Screening

Screening has not yet proved beneficial in patients with lung cancer.

Symptoms at presentation

- Cough
- Haemoptysis
- Chest pain
- Recurrent chest infection
- Hoarseness
- Breathlessness
- Tiredness
- Pancoast syndrome and Horner syndrome (damaged sympathetic eye nerves, causing miosis, ptosis, and loss of hemifacial sweating)

> ### Stop and Think
>
> Why do many Western societies have so much enthusiasm for expensive cancer screening programmes, and yet provide so little support for those wishing to stop smoking?

Diagnosis and staging

Diagnosis

- Chest X-ray
- Chest computerized tomography (CT) scan
- Sputum cytology
- Bronchial brushings and washings
- Bronchoscopy with biopsy
- CT guided biopsy

- Mediastinoscopy or video-assisted thoracoscopy with biopsy
- Pleural effusion cytology

Staging

- Bronchoscopy
- CT scan of chest and abdomen
- Mediastinoscopy
- Pleural effusion cytology, pleural biopsy
- Bone and brain scan if symptomatic
- Positron emission tomography scan for mediastinal nodes and distant metastases (if resectability uncertain)
- Magnetic resonance imaging for apical lesions (to define relation to nerves and vessels if surgery is considered)

Non-metastatic paraneoplastic syndromes

Between 10 and 20% of patients may present with, or develop complications of, the non-metastatic paraneoplastic syndromes associated with lung cancer. These are particularly well documented for small cell carcinoma and large cell undifferentiated carcinoma, both of which tend to have many neuroendocrine features. However, they do occur to a lesser degree with squamous cell carcinoma and adenocarcinoma. Many of these syndromes are mediated by peptides, which mimic active portions of known hormones.

Small cell lung cancer (SCLC)

This is generally believed to be a systemic disease at the time of diagnosis and thus surgery plays no part in the management of this disease.

SCLC staging

Limited disease – confined to one hemithorax that can be included in a reasonable field of thoracic radiation therapy.

Extensive disease – present beyond one hemithorax or that cannot be included in a reasonable field of thoracic radiation therapy.

SCLC management

- Because of chemoresponsiveness and frequent dissemination at diagnosis, combination chemotherapy is the treatment of choice

TABLE 8.1 Paraneoplastic syndromes and their clinical effects

Paraneoplastic syndrome	Clinical effect
Endocrine	
Syndrome of inappropriate antidiuretic hormone (SIADH)	Dehydration, low plasma sodium
Atrial natriuretic peptide	Dehydration
Ectopic adrenocorticotropic hormone	Cushing's syndrome, low potassium,
	hyperpigmentation, glucose intolerance
Hypercalcaemia (non-metastatic)	Thirst, vomiting, confusion, constipation
Neurological	
Eaton–Lambert myasthenic syndrome	Weakness in shoulder and pelvic girdle muscles
Paraneoplastic cerebellar degeneration	Unsteady gait, ataxia, vertigo, diplopia
Encephalomyelitis	Confusion, memory loss, agitation
Sensory neuropathy	Pain and limb paraesthesia
Retinopathy	Visual disturbance
Intestinal pseudo-obstruction	Bloating and constipation
Autonomic dysfunction	Hypotension
Other	
Hypercoagulability	Venous thrombosis
Nephrotic syndrome	Hypoproteinemia, oedema

- Many chemotherapeutic agents have demonstrated activity in this disease. Commonly used regimens include cisplatin/etoposide and cyclophosphamide/doxorubicin/vincristine

- For patients with limited stage disease, thoracic irradiation in addition to chemotherapy improves local disease control and prolongs survival in patients who have a good response to chemotherapy when compared with chemotherapy alone. Prophylactic cranial irradiation reduces the incidence of brain metastases but has not been shown to prolong survival

- Radiotherapy may be a useful palliative treatment for patients relapsing after, or resistant to, chemotherapy, or when they develop metastases

Prognosis

- Approximately 80% of patients respond to chemotherapy but the majority relapse and only 10% of patients are alive 2 years following diagnosis

Non-small cell lung cancer (NSCLC)

NSCLC metastasizes later in its course than SCLC and consequently surgery offers the best chance of cure. All patients being considered for surgical treatment must be thoroughly staged to determine tumour resectability. PET will help to assess regional nodal involvement and distant metastases. Unfortunately only 15% of patients are suitable for resection at diagnosis.[3] The patient must also be carefully assessed pre-operatively to assure fitness for surgery.

Post-operative mortality rate should be less than 5% (British Thoracic Society Guidelines[4]).

NSCLC management

Surgery

Surgical resection offers the best chance of cure in this disease. The aim is to resect the primary tumour with clear margins along with the draining peribronchial and hilar lymph nodes. Mediastinal lymph nodes are also resected or sampled.

Lobectomy is the most commonly performed operation but a bilobectomy or pneumonectomy may be performed for more extensive tumours.

Conversely, in less fit patients with limited respiratory reserve only a partial lobectomy may be tolerated although the results from this surgery in terms of the risk of tumour recurrence may be inferior. In selected patients, smaller resections can be done through the thoracoscope with less post-operative pain.

TABLE 8.2 TNM staging of lung cancer

T_1	Tumour < 3 cm diameter; distal to main bronchus
T_2	Tumour > 3 cm diameter; or involving main bronchus 2 cm distal to carina; or invading visceral pleura; or atelectasis extending to hilum
T_3	Tumour invading chest wall, diaphragm, mediastinal pleura or pericardium; or tumour in main bronchus < 2 cm distal to carina or atelectasis of whole lung
T_4	Tumour invading mediastinum, heart, major vessels, trachea, oesophagus, vertebra or carina; or separate tumour nodules in the same lobe; or malignant pleural effusion
N_0	No regional node metastases
N_1	Ipsilateral peribronchial or hilar nodes
N_2	Ipsilateral mediastinal or subcarinal nodes
N_3	Contralateral mediastinal nodes; scalene or supraclavicular nodes
M_1	Distant metastasis present, including separate tumour nodule(s) in a different lobe (ipsilateral or contralateral)

TABLE 8.3	Stages and groupings used in lung cancer

Stage	Grouping
I	$T_{1-2} N_0$
II	$T_{1-2} N_1$ or $T_3 N_0$
IIIa	$T_{1-2} N_2$ or $T_3 N_{1-2}$
IIIb	T_4 any N M_0 or any T $N_3 M_0$
IV	Any T any N M_1

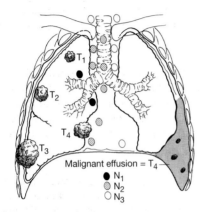

Fig. 8.1 NSCLC, tumour and node staging.

Radiotherapy
Radical radiotherapy
Selected patients with stage I–III disease who are unfit for surgery or patients with unresectable stage III disease may be suitable for radical radiotherapy. Induction chemotherapy to downstage the tumour can be considered in these patients. Five-year survival of 15–20% has been reported in this highly selected patient group.

The benefit of adjuvant thoracic radiotherapy following surgery for high-risk disease is uncertain but may reduce the risk of local disease relapse.

Palliative radiotherapy
Radiotherapy is a key component of symptomatic treatment for:

◆ Haemoptysis

◆ Chest pain

◆ Breathlessness due to bronchial occlusion

◆ Pain from bone metastasis

◆ Symptoms from brain metastasis

Chemotherapy
NSCLC is much less chemosensitive than SCLC. In patients with good performance status (ECOG Performance Scale 0–1) and advanced NSCLC (stage IV and selected IIIb), platinum-based therapy improves quality of life and survival in the palliative setting. Commonly used regimens include cisplatin/paclitaxel, cisplatin/vinorelbine, cisplatin/gemcitabine, mitomycin C/ifosfamide/cisplatin.

Patients with less good performance status and/or elderly patients (age > 70 years) with advanced NSCLC may benefit from palliative single-agent chemotherapy, such as vinorelbine or gemcitabine.

Second-line chemotherapy is not widely used, but single agent docetaxel or pemetrexed improves survival and quality of life in selected patients with good performance status and progressive disease following treatment with a platinum-based regimen.

The epidermal growth factor receptor tyrosine kinase inhibitor erlotinib is active in advanced NSCLC, with a higher chance of response in female patients, non-smokers, those of Asian origin, and adenocarcinoma/bronchiolo-alveolar histology. Although response rates are low, a higher proportion of patients gain symptomatic benefit and there is a modest improvement in survival in previously treated patients.

Chemotherapy may also be used in the neoadjuvant setting to down-stage a tumour prior to consideration of radical surgery or radiation therapy, mostly in patients with stage III disease. Adjuvant platinum-based chemotherapy following radical surgery also confers a modest survival benefit.

Specific issues
Because most patients present with advanced disease, the prognosis is usually very poor (Table 8.4). This and the link to smoking may cause particular distress. Lung cancers often occur in association with pre-existing

TABLE 8.4	Prognosis of NSCLC

Stage	Five-year survival
I	60–80%
II	25–40%
IIIa	10–15%
IIIb	3–7%
IV	1%

Test Yourself

How would you differentiate between symptoms associated with smoking and symptoms of lung cancer?

lung disease which may alter the patient's perception of breathlessness or cough and delay diagnosis.

Specific pain issues

- **Pleuritic pain** may be associated with the tumour itself, metastases in ribs, or local inflammation. This type of pain responds well to non-steroidal anti-inflammatory drugs. It may also be helped by local nerve blockade in addition to radiotherapy

- **Pancoast tumours (pleural and chest wall spread associated with Horner's syndrome together with brachial plexus invasion)** can produce severe neuropathic pain which may only be partially opioid responsive and will need adjuvant analgesics* such as amitriptyline or gabapentin. Early referral for specialist help

- **Bone metastases** may occur, putting the patient at risk of pathological fractures and spinal cord compression. Emergency surgery or radiotherapy may be needed. Specialist advice from orthopaedics, clinical oncology or palliative medicine should be sought

Other complications

Breathlessness

This is common and can be very distressing for carers. Reversible causes such as anaemia and pleural effusion should be treated where appropriate. Pleurodesis to prevent re-accumulation of fluid may be appropriate in selected patients. Clear explanations of what is happening should be given. Practical measures such as sitting upright, opening windows, and using fans should be discussed with the patient and family. Selected patients may benefit from oxygen supplementation.

Regular doses of short-acting oral morphine every 2–4 hours may decrease the sensation of breathlessness. Other more specialist interventions such as palliative radiotherapy, endobronchial laser therapy, and stenting may help some patients. Panic and anxiety are

---

*An adjuvant analgesic is a drug that is not an analgesic in its prime function but that in combination with an analgesic can enhance pain control, for example an anxiolytic.

frequently associated with breathlessness and may be helped by simple relaxation techniques. A low dose of an anxiolytic such as diazepam may be helpful. Nebulized opioids have been used for breathlessness but are no more effective than inhaled saline.

Cough

Cough can exacerbate breathlessness and pain, and affect sleep and a patient's ability to eat. Its management will depend on the cause but it is often appropriate to try to suppress the cough pharmacologically using codeine or morphine linctus. If not responding to simple measures refer to palliative care team or breathlessness clinic.

Altered taste and anorexia

These are common and often treatment-related. Good oral hygiene and effective treatment of oral candidiasis may help. Carers may find it helpful to talk through different ways of encouraging the patient to eat, such as supplement drinks, frequent small meals, etc.

Haemoptysis

Haemoptysis is a frightening symptom. Palliative radiotherapy may be effective if the patient is fit. Oral anti-fibrinolytics such as tranexamic acid may also help. Occasionally frequent small episodes herald a catastrophic haemoptysis. This is rare, but is a very difficult situation to manage at home. The risks of frightening a family with information about a possible risk of catastrophic haemoptysis need to be balanced against the potential distress that could be caused by leaving a patient and family unprepared. Rarely angiography and embolization may be required in carefully selected patients.

Hypercalcaemia

Hypercalcaemia may occur. It should be considered in any patient with persistent nausea, thirst, altered mood or confusion (even if intermittent), worsening pain, and/or constipation. It should be treated with intravenous hydration and bisphosphonates unless the patient is clearly dying, in which case treatment is not appropriate.

Cerebral metastases

Cerebral metastases are common. Decisions about investigation and management may be complex and need to be made on an individual basis. Persistent headache, worse in the mornings, and unexplained vomiting are early signs of this diagnosis. Altered behaviour and personality as well as problems of comprehension and communication can be very distressing for relatives. There is a risk of epileptic fits and prophylactic anti-convulsant medication is appropriate following the first epileptic fit.

Hyponatraemia

Hyponatraemia and other biochemical imbalances are particularly common in SCLC. Management can be complex and advice may be required from the metabolic team.

Superior vena cava obstruction

This can occur, particularly in patients with right-sided lung and centrally located cancers. Management includes consideration of vascular stenting, radiotherapy, and high-dose oral steroids.

Mesothelioma

General comments

This usually affects the pleura but can affect other mesothelial linings, most commonly the peritoneum. It is associated with exposure to asbestos although the history may be difficult to elicit because the risk of mesothelioma appears unrelated to the length of exposure to asbestos and may occur many years after such exposure. Ninety per cent of cases are men with the mean age at diagnosis being 64 years.

The use of asbestos was banned gradually from the mid-1960s. As there is a lag time from the date of first exposure until the diagnosis of mesothelioma, the incidence is expected to rise for a further 15 years in Western Europe, peaking in 2020.

The mean lag time from first asbestos contact to diagnosis is 40 years, though it is shorter for insulation workers, suggesting a dose–response relationship.

It is important that the patient is aware that they and their families may be entitled to *compensation* and should consult a specialist lawyer about this.

Key Fact

All deaths from mesothelioma should be discussed with the coroner, who will most probably carry out a post-mortem unless the disease was clearly not related to industrial exposure or a tissue diagnosis has already been made. The family should be forewarned that the coroner will be contacted (regardless of any compensation claims or litigation), to try to minimize distress at the time of death.

Diagnosis

- Chest X-ray
- CT scan of chest
- Mediastinoscopy or thoracoscopy with pleural biopsy

There is a high incidence of false negative biopsies – in some cases these may need to be repeated a number of times to make a diagnosis.

Treatment

Surgery

Radical surgery is of uncertain value with a high mortality and few long-term survivors reported.

Palliative surgery with parietal pleurectomy and decortication of the lung may offer palliation with minimal morbidity.

Radiotherapy

The tumour may grow along the track of a biopsy or drainage needle to produce a cutaneous lesion. These areas can become painful, and ulcerated and can be difficult to manage.

Radiotherapy is given prophylactically following the biopsy. It may also be used locally for established cutaneous spread.

Chemotherapy

The value of chemotherapy in mesothelioma is uncertain. Recent reports, however, suggest that selected patients may respond to the combination of platinum and pemetrexed with some palliative benefit.

Specific problems in the management of patients with mesothelioma

- **Pleural effusions** are common, frequently blood-stained, and become increasingly difficult to aspirate as the disease progresses. *Pleurodesis* to prevent re-accumulation of fluid may be helpful if carried out early

- **Breathlessness** can be severe when pleural disease reduces the capacity of the lung or when there is a pleural effusion. Clear explanations of what is happening must be given to patients and their families. Ensure that practical measures such as sitting the patient up, opening windows, and using fans have been discussed with the patient and family. Selected patients may benefit from oxygen supplementation. *Regular doses of short acting oral morphine* every 2–4 hours may decrease the sensation of breathlessness. A low dose of an *anxiolytic* such as diazepam may be helpful. Other treatment options are limited

◆ **Ascites** occurs with peritoneal mesothelioma. The ascitic fluid is frequently blood-stained and becomes increasingly difficult to aspirate as the disease progresses

Specific pain complexes

◆ Mesotheliomas can produce severe neuropathic pain which will only be partially opioid responsive and will need adjuvant analgesics. Early referral to the palliative care team should be considered. Local nerve blockades can help in some cases

CASE HISTORY

A woman with NSCLC

A 65-year-old asymptomatic woman accompanied her sister to a consultation with her GP. The doctor noticed that her fingers were 'clubbed' (Fig. 8.2) and arranged a chest X-ray. This showed a right upper lobe tumour occupying nearly half the right lung (Fig. 8.3). On bronchoscopy, tumour was seen protruding from the right upper lobe orifice into the right main bronchus (Fig. 8.4); biopsy showed this to be poorly differentiated squamous carcinoma. CT scan showed a bulky tumour with maximum diameter 15 cm, abutting the chest wall laterally and the mediastinum medially, surrounding the hilum on the right side

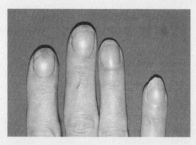

Fig. 8.2 Finger clubbing.

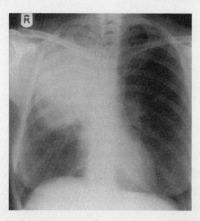

Fig. 8.3 Pre-chemotherapy chest X-ray.

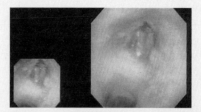

Fig. 8.4 The right upper lobe bronchus is occluded by tumour.

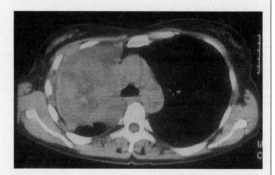

Fig. 8.5 Pre-chemotherapy CT scan.

(Fig. 8.5) (the hilum is not clearly evaluable in the CT scan image in Fig. 8.5). There was no evidence of distant metastases.

Surgical opinion was that the tumour was unresectable but would be considered for surgery if there was significant tumour shrinkage after induction therapy.

After two courses of uncomplicated 'MIC' chemotherapy (Mitomycin C® 6 mg/m², ifosfamide 3 g/m², and cisplatin 50 mg/m²), there was noticeable tumour shrinkage.

After the fourth course (the mitomycin was witheld from the last course to reduce side effects on the lung), there remained a 5 cm necrotic mass well clear of the chest wall and mediastinum. At surgery there was a 5 cm mass restricted to the upper lobe but thickened tissue around the main bronchus and in the lower paratracheal nodes. Right pneumonectomy was performed with clearance of ipsilateral mediastinal lymph

---

nodes (Fig. 8.6). Pathology showed no residual tumour cells (pathological complete response). Twenty-four hours later there was evidence of acute post-pneumonectomy lung injury in the remaining lung. This was successfully treated with diuretics, intensive chest physiotherapy, and a minitracheostomy (cricothyroidotomy to remove secretions).

Four and a half years later the patient is alive with no evidence of recurrent disease. She lives independently and provides day care for her new granddaughter. The finger clubbing remains; it may have been congenital, although reversal after successful treatment does not always occur.

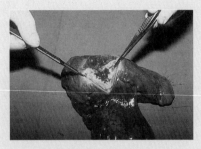

Fig. 8.6 Following pneumonectomy a 5-cm necrotic tumour is seen in the right upper lobe.

Chapter summary

- Most common cancer in men and women in UK and USA
- 80% due to smoking
- Small cell lung cancer (SCLC) 25%
- Non-small cell lung cancer (NSCLC) 75%
  - Squamous cell carcinoma 30%
  - Adenocarcinoma 35%
  - Large cell anaplastic 10%

SCLC

- This is generally believed to be a systemic disease at the time of diagnosis
- Because of chemo-responsiveness and frequent dissemination at diagnosis combination chemotherapy is the treatment of choice
- Approximately 80% of patients respond to chemotherapy but the majority relapse and only approximately 10% of patients are alive 2 years following diagnosis

NSCLC

- Metastasizes later in its course than SCLC and consequently surgery offers the best chance of cure when tumour is resectable at diagnosis
- Selected patients with stage I–III disease who are unfit for surgery may be suitable for radical radiotherapy

- Radiotherapy is a key component of symptomatic treatment for
  - Haemoptysis
  - Chest pain
  - Dyspnoea
  - Cough
  - Pain from bone metastasis
  - Symptoms from brain metastasis
- Although NSCLC is much less chemosensitive than SCLC, chemotherapy can improve survival and quality of life in patients with NSCLC

Mesothelioma

- The risk of mesothelioma does not appear to be directly correlated to the length of exposure to asbestos and it may occur many years after such exposure. There may be a relationship to the intensity of exposure
- Radical surgery is of uncertain value with a high mortality, and few long-term survivors are reported
- Chemotherapy provides useful palliation in selected patients
- Mesotheliomas can produce severe neuropathic pain which will only be partially opioid responsive and will need adjuvant analgesics

References

1. http://info.cancerresearchuk.org/cancerstats/incidence/commoncancers/
2. http://info.cancerresearchuk.org/images/excel/cs_mort_f1.1.xls
3. http://www.cancerresearchuk.org/aboutus/publications/scientific_yearbook/researcharticles/lung_cancer.pdf
4. British Thoracic Society: Society of Cardiothoracic Surgeons of Great Britain and Ireland Working Party. BTS guidelines: guidelines on the selection of patients with lung cancer for surgery. *Thorax* 2001, **56**, 89–108.

Case studies and multiple choice questions at
www.oxfordtextbooks.co.uk/orc/watson/

Patients with colorectal cancer

Incidence and mortality

In 2001 18,500 men and 16,000 women were diagnosed with colorectal cancer in the UK.[1]

In 2003 8,500 men and 7,500 women died from colorectal cancer in the UK.[2]

Background

- Third commonest cancer in the UK: fourth commonest worldwide
- In the UK approximately 13% of all new cancers diagnosed are colorectal
- Approximately 50% of tumours occur in the rectum or sigmoid colon
- Majority occur in the over 50 age group
- Peak incidence 60–80 years
- Dietary factors are thought to be important
- Tumour may be nodular, ulcerating, or polypoid in appearance.
- Vast majority are adenocarcinoma with 20% being mucinous in type
- Tumour often secretes the oncofetal antigen carcino-embryonic antigen (CEA)
- 6–8% of cases are familial
- Associated syndromes include familial adenomatous polyposis coli and hereditary non-polyposis coli

Natural history

TABLE 9.1   Risk factors associated with colorectal cancer

Familial
Familial adenomatous polyposis
Gardner syndrome
Hetediatry non-polyposis colorectal cancer (Lynch I & II)
Dietary
High intake of red meat and animal fat
Low intake of dietary fibre
Risk reduced by ingestion of aspirin or other non-steroidal anti-inflammatory agents
Colorectal disease
Previous colorectal cancer
Ulcerative colitis
Crohn's disease of colon
Ureteric diversion to sigmoid colon
Previous cholecystectomy

Key Facts

Colorectal cancer

- 50 % of tumours are within reach of a sigmoidoscope (rectum and sigmoid colon)
- Above the level of the rectum, large bowel cancers are now thought to be evenly distributed throughout the whole length of the colon
- Most cancers represent malignant change in a benign adenomatous polyp

Stop and Think

'I'm Loving it!'
Will McDonald's® salad meals change the incidence of colorectal cancer?

Examination

With 33% of colorectal tumours within the rectum the importance of a rectal examination in patients present-

TABLE 9.2   Characteristic clinical patterns of colorectal cancer presentation

Acute large bowel obstruction (20%)	Left-sided tumour
Anaemia and palpable abdominal mass (15%)	Right-sided tumour
Rectal irritation and bleeding (33%)	Rectal tumour
Change in bowel habit (especially alternation of diarrhoea and constipation)	

Key Facts

Dukes' staging
The traditional staging system for colorectal carcinoma was Dukes':

A – Confined to mucosa and submucosa
B – Penetrated muscularis mucosa
C – Regional lymph node involvement
D – Distant metastases

This has been modified several times to the point where the Dukes' system has been undermined.

At presentation around 5% tumours are Dukes' A and roughly equal numbers are B, C, and D.

ing with bowel symptoms must be stressed. 'If you don't put your finger in, you will put your foot in it.'

Screening

There is increasing evidence that, although expensive, a screening programme can allow the diagnosis of colorectal cancer while still at Dukes' A or B stage. This may lead to a significant survival advantage for the screened population. This is commencing in England and Wales in 2007. See earlier section on screening in Chapter 1.

Staging and diagnosis

- Colonoscopy – all patients should have full evaluation of the colon prior to surgery
- Sigmoidoscopy
- Barium enema (with the advent of colonoscopy this is used less frequently)
- Computerized tomography (CT)
  - Staging CT
  - Virtual colonoscopy (CT colonography). This test creates a three-dimensional reconstruction of the colonic wall

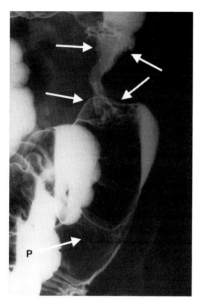

Fig. 9.1 Barium enema: carcinoma of descending colon with 'apple core' lesion arrowed, and a synchronous polyp in the distal descending colon labelled 'P'.

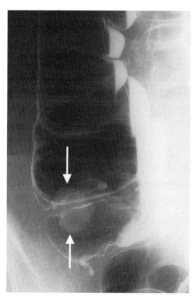

Fig. 9.2 Barium enema: polypoid tumour 'arrowed' in the caecum of a patient presenting with iron deficiency anaemia.

Key Fact

The stage of colorectal cancer is usually quoted as a number I, II, III, IV derived from the TNM system grouped by prognosis; a higher number indicates a more advanced cancer and a probable worse outcome.

- Magnetic resonance imaging (MRI)/endorectal ultrasound are important to assess local extent of tumour in the rectum
- Positron emission tomography scan has a role in defining the significance of radiological abnormalities after surgery/radiotherapy to demonstrate distal spread

Selected features associated with adverse prognosis on pathological examination

Lymph node features:

- Presence and number of involved lymph nodes
- Lack of lymphocytic response to tumour
- Lymphovascular invasion

Tumour margin features:

- Depth of presentation through the layers of bowel wall
- Involvement of the circumferential resection margin (especially relevant for rectal cancer)
- Infiltrating rather than pushing tumour edge

Other features:

- Mucinous cell type
- Venous invasion
- Perineural invasion

TABLE 9.3	TNM staging for colorectal cancer
T_{is}	Carcinoma *in situ*
T_1	Invades submucosa
T_2	Invades muscularis propria
T_3	Invades subserosa
T_4	Invades through serosa
N_0	No lymph node involvement
N_1	One to three nodes involved
N_2	Four or more nodes involved
N_3	Central nodes involved
M_0	No distant metastases
M_1	Distant metastases

STAGE 0

T_{is} N_0 M_0

Tumour is small in size, non-invasive and limited to the inside lining of the colon or rectum

Likely treatment: surgery

STAGE I

T_1 N_0 M_0 or

T_2 N_0 M_0

Tumour has moved into other layers of the colon, without spreading beyond the wall

Likely treatment: surgery

STAGE II

T_3 N_0 M_0 or

T_4 N_0 M_0

Tumour has gone through the wall of the colon or rectum, affecting nearby tissue, without affecting lymph nodes

Likely treatment: surgery, chemotherapy, radiation therapy (rectal cancer)

STAGE III

T_1 N_1 M_0

T_2 N_1 M_0

T_3 N_1 M_0

Any T N_2 M_0

Tumour has spread to nearby lymph nodes, but not to other organs

Possible treatment: surgery, chemotherapy, radiation therapy

STAGE IV

Any T Any N M_1

Tumour has spread to other organs and/or tissues such as liver and lungs

Likely treatment: surgery, chemotherapy, radiation therapy (rectal cancer), targeted therapy

Fig. 9.3 TNM staging for colorectal cancer.

Management

Surgery

Surgery of primary disease

Surgery is the mainstay of therapy for colorectal cancer. For colonic tumours a segment of colon with its blood supply and draining nodes is excised. Depending on the site of the tumour this may involve a right or left hemicolectomy or a sigmoid colectomy. Surgery is usually carried out by laparotomy, but in selected patients laparoscopic resection is favoured.

Rectal cancer surgery is difficult and technically challenging. Traditionally, surgery for lower rectal tumours has involved an abdomino-perineal approach but in many cases this can be avoided. In the past, without radiotherapy local relapse rates of 25–30% have been reported. Traditionally, radiotherapy has been used post-operatively but increasingly chemo-radiotherapy is being used to 'sterilize' the area prior to surgery. Local recurrence rates are much lower (< 10%) using the modern surgical technique of total mesorectal excision (TME), where the rectum is excised en bloc with the adjacent perirectal tissue. With TME the role of chemo-radiotherapy is less clear, although it is still valuable where the resection margins are involved.

Surgery for hepatic metastases

In the majority of patients, the liver is the first site of disease progression. A proportion of these patients may be suitable for metastatectomy, often after initial chemotherapy. Up to 40% 5-year survival has been reported for carefully selected patients. Radiofrequency ablation of colorectal liver secondaries is showing promise.

Chemotherapy

Adjuvant chemotherapy of colorectal cancer

Large randomized controlled trials have shown a clear survival advantage with 5-fluorouracil-based or capecitabine therapy for patients with lymph node involvement, 5-year survival rates increasing from 64 to 71%.[3] The addition of oxoliplatin to 5-fluorouracil further improves survival.

For Dukes' B (T_2–T_4) the trials are less conclusive, but increasingly chemotherapy is offered to such patients.

TABLE 9.4 Surgery for liver metastases from colorectal cancer

Diagnostic investigations
Transabdominal and intra-operative ultrasound
Contrast enhanced CT scan
CT with arterial portography
Pre-resection laparoscopy
Bimanual assessment at laparotomy
Indications for surgery
No extrahepatic metastatic disease
Limited number of lesions
Outcome
2% mortality
16–40% 5-year survival

Advanced colorectal cancer

5-Fluorouracil-based chemotherapy also confers a benefit in patients with metastatic disease. There appears to be a survival advantage with chemotherapy of at least 6 months, increasing survival from approximately 6 to 12 months. Capecitabine is an orally available prodrug of 5-fluorouracil that is as active as 5-fluorouracil but more convenient and better tolerated.

The addition of oxaliplatin or irinotecan to 5 fluorouracil further prolongs survival to around 18 months. Survival appears best in patients who receive each of the cytotoxics during the course of their disease.

Biological therapy

This is a new approach, but one with considerable potential. The anti-vascular endothelial growth factor (VEGF) monoclonal antibody bevacizumab 'mops up' circulating VEGF and adds to the efficacy of chemotherapy in colorectal cancer, further prolonging survival. Another monoclonal antibody, cetuximab, targets the epidermal growth factor receptor and enhances the activity of irinotecan. Both monoclonal antibodies are expensive and their optimal use has yet to be defined. Nevertheless their use is likely to increase in the next few years.

Radiotherapy

Radiotherapy is not routinely given in colon cancer.

Adjuvant treatment

Pelvic radiotherapy with concurrent fluoropyrimidine chemotherapy reduces the risk of pelvic relapse for patients with Dukes' stage B and C rectal cancer (T_2–N_3).

Pelvic chemo-radiotherapy may also be useful for patients with large fixed rectal tumours to reduce tumour volume prior to consideration of surgical resection.

TABLE 9.5 Prognosis

	5-year survival
Dukes' A (T1)	> 90%
Dukes' B1 (T2)	> 80%
Dukes' B2 (T3)	> 50%
Dukes' C	30–40%

Advanced disease

Radiotherapy may be used to palliate local recurrence of rectal cancer within the pelvis.

Symptomatic management of patients with advanced disease

- **Liver metastases** often occur and may cause capsular pain. This usually responds well to non-steroidal anti-inflammatory drugs or steroids. Liver metastases may also lead to hepatomegaly causing squashed stomach syndrome with delayed gastric emptying and a feeling of fullness. This may respond to a pro-kinetic agent such as metoclopramide

- **Perineal and pelvic pain** may be caused by advancing disease or may be iatrogenic. There is nearly always a neuropathic element to the pain, which will only be partially opioid sensitive. Tenesmus is a unique type of neuropathic pain which may require intervention by palliative care doctors or anaesthetists

- **Bowel obstruction**, unless it can be palliated surgically, should be managed medically using a syringe driver containing a mixture of analgesics, anti-emetics, and anti-spasmodics
  Multiple levels of obstruction of the bowel, which is a not infrequent situation, may make surgery inappropriate. Differentiating between a high blockage (where vomiting is a feature) and blockage lower in the bowel can be useful in targeting treatment strategies. Imaging techniques may also be helpful to delineate the level of obstruction. Sometimes a short segment in the colon may be amenable to colonic stenting via endoscopy

- **Fistulae** between the bowel and the skin or bladder may occur. These can be very difficult to manage and require a multidisciplinary approach with specialist input

- **Rectal discharge and bleeding** are unpleasant and difficult symptoms to manage. Referral to a clinical oncologist is appropriate as radiotherapy may be of benefit. After a colostomy the blind loop rectal stump may continue to discharge

- **Hypoproteinaemia** is common because of poor oral intake and poor absorption from the bowel and may lead to lower limb oedema

- **Poor appetite** is not uncommon and can be helped with the use of steroids.

Bowel stomata

A bowel stoma is an artificial opening, created surgically, for patients to allow faeces to leave the body by a new route through a spout or outlet on the abdomen. The majority of stomata have been fashioned following surgical resection for a low rectal cancer or as a bypass for inoperable or recurrent cancers of the bowel (or ovary) causing obstruction. Bowel stomata are generally created from the colon (colostomy) or ileum (ileostomy). The bowel proximal to the stoma continues to function in the normal way whereas function distal to this is normally lost.

Temporary (de-functioning) stomata

These include loop ileostomies or colostomies which are usually created to protect an anastomosis or to facilitate decompression or healing in the distal bowel. The proximal opening allows the passage of stool which is collected in a stoma bag and the distal opening leads to the redundant section of bowel. Mucus and old faeces may be expelled through the rectum.

Permanent stomata

These are end sections of bowel which are brought to the skin surface. The potential stoma site along the path of the bowel is planned preoperatively, if possible, to allow optimal positioning of a stoma bag for the individual. The stoma nurse is invaluable in counselling and advising patients.

@ Case studies and multiple choice questions at www.oxfordtextbooks.co.uk/orc/watson/

Test Yourself

JH: Rectal adenocarcinoma

GP surgery

A 72-year-old farmer, JH, presented to his GP having noticed a small amount of rectal bleeding. Examination revealed that JH had haemorrhoids and his GP prescribed ointment but advised that if the bleeding did not settle he should return.

Five weeks later JH returned to the surgery complaining that the bleeding had worsened and that he had also noticed a rectal discharge. On rectal examination the GP was suspicious that he could feel a craggy mass in the anterior rectal wall. He therefore arranged an urgent appointment with the local colorectal surgeon.

Colorectal surgeon and clinical oncologist

Sigmoidoscopy confirmed the presence of a rectal tumour and the biopsy report showed moderately differentiated adenocarcinoma.

Barium enema showed no other lesion in the large bowel.

Chest X-ray showed no evidence of metastases. CT scan of abdomen and pelvis showed no evidence of extension outside the colon, of lymph nodes or liver metastases.

The CEA was 7 µg/l (normal < 4 µg/l) and liver function tests were normal.

MRI and transrectal ultrasound did not reveal extension of tumour beyond the bowel wall but there was a suspicion of lymph node involvement.

1. How would you stage JH's rectal tumour?

Following multidisciplinary discussion JH received neoadjuvant radiotherapy to the rectum and the lymphatic drainage area of the rectum.

One week later JH underwent surgery with removal of the tumour (TME), and immediate re-anastomosis.

Pathology

Pathology confirmed moderately differentiated adenocarcinoma which had penetrated through the full thickness of the bowel wall but the resection margins were fully clear of tumour. Two lymph nodes were involved, and there was venous invasion.

2. How would you designate JH's tumour according to the Dukes' classification? Why is this designation important?

Medical oncologist

JH received 6 months of adjuvant 5-fluorouracil/folinic acid. He was followed up monthly for 6 months, then 3-monthly, then 6-monthly. After 2 years at routine follow-up the CEA was noted to have risen to 24. On rechecking, this result was confirmed. This initiated re-staging even though JH was feeling well and had returned to active life on his farm.

3. What investigations would you order for re-staging at this time?

The results revealed a large solitary metastasis in the left lobe of the liver. No other area of active disease was diagnosed.

JH was referred to a hepatic surgeon and a resection of the left lobe of his liver was carried out, from which he recovered uneventfully.

The CEA returned to normal after surgery and has remained so on routine review for the past 3½ years.

Chapter summary

- Third commonest cancer in the UK, fourth commonest worldwide

- Peak incidence 60–80 years

- 6–8% of cases are familial

- 50% of tumours are within reach of a sigmoidoscope (rectum and sigmoid colon)

- The most common screening tool is faecal occult blood testing

- Surgery is the mainstay of therapy for colorectal cancer

- Total mesorectal excision (TME) surgery has significantly reduced local recurrence rates in patients with rectal cancer

- The commonest first site of disease progression is the liver

- A proportion of patients may be suitable for hepatic or pulmonary metastatectomy or formal anatomical liver resection. Up to 40% 5-year survival has been reported for carefully selected patients

- Adjuvant chemotherapy with 5-fluorouracil-based therapy for patients with lymph node involvement has shown a clear survival advantage

- For Dukes' B tumours the clinical trials are less conclusive, but chemotherapy may have a small survival benefit

- Pelvic radiotherapy with concurrent chemotherapy reduces risk of pelvic relapse for patients with Dukes' stage B and C rectal cancer

- Palliative chemotherapy prolongs survival; the best results are seen in patients exposed to each of the active agents

- The role of biological therapies is likely to increase

References

1. http://info.cancerresearchuk.org/cancerstats/incidence/commoncancers/
2. http://info.cancerresearchuk.org/images/excel/cs_mort_f1.1.xls
3. Sargent, DJ *et al.* A pooled analysis of adjuvant chemotherapy for resected colon cancer in elderly patients. *New England Journal of Medicine* 2001, **345**, 1091–1097.

CHAPTER 10

Patients with breast cancer

Chapter contents

Incidence and mortality

In 2001 294 men and 41,000 women were diagnosed with breast cancer in the UK.[1]

In 2003 82 men and 12,600 women died from breast cancer in the UK.[2]

Background

- Accounts for 20% of all cancers in Western Europe and the USA

- Life time risk for women is 1 in 9

- For most women a specific cause of their breast cancer is not known

- Factors which increase the risk of breast cancer include increasing age, a family history of breast cancer, nulliparity, early menarche and late menopause, use of hormone replacement therapy (HRT), and the contraceptive pill

- Incidence of breast cancer is increasing although overall mortality is decreasing (Stage I 80% 5 year survival)

- Breast cancer is diagnosed more frequently in affluent women, but prognosis (i.e. survival) is worse for those who are socially deprived

- Male breast cancer is rare – accounting for only 0.7% of all breast cancers

- The pathological findings in the axilla are used to asign the N stage (pM) in breast cancer

TABLE 10.1	Risk factors for breast cancer
Factor	**Estimated relative risk**
Increased age	15
Geographical location	6
Early age at menarche	2
Late age of menopause	3
Age at first birth greater than 32 years	4
Nulliparity	4
Obesity	3
Alcohol intake	1.2
Irradiation	5
Oral contraceptive	1.84
HRT	1.36
Benign disease:	
Atypical ductal hyperplasia	5
Sclerosing adenosis	1.5
Family history in first-degree relatives	8

Pathology of breast carcinoma

Preinvasive lesion

- Lobular carcinoma *in situ* (LCIS) – an indication of risk which needs follow-up
- Ductal carcinoma *in situ* (DCIS) – usually detected mammographically, may progress to invasive disease and need excision, often after localization

Key Fact

Tumour cells cannot spread until they penetrate the basement membrane and come into contact with lymphatics and blood vessels. Hence *in situ* tumour cells (which have not yet crossed the basement membrane) cannot spread until they become 'invasive'.

Invasive lesion

- Ductal carcinoma 80%
- Lobular carcinoma 10%
- Medullary carcinoma 5%
- Tubular carcinoma 2%

Genetics of breast cancer

Between 5 and 10% of breast cancers are believed to be hereditary. Many of these cancers are the result of germline mutations in the tumour suppressor genes *BRCA1* or *BRCA2*. For patients with proven mutations in the *BRCA1* or *BRCA2* gene prophylactic bilateral subcutaneous mastectomy, often with reconstruction, reduces the incidence of breast cancer by 95%. At present, treatment for a breast tumour arising in a mutation carrier is the same as for non-mutation carriers.

Key Fact

A genetic basis for breast cancer is suspected when a woman diagnosed with breast cancer has a family history of breast or ovarian cancer, especially when these diagnoses were made in relatively young relatives (<40 years).

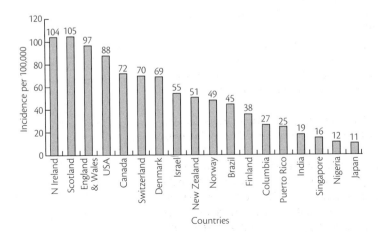

Fig. 10.1 Geographical variation in incidence of breast cancer.

Stop and Think

Female population risk for breast cancer age 40–50 years is 1 in 100 (1%).

Female population lifetime risk aged 20–80 is 1 in 9 (11 %).

Screening for breast cancer (also see screening section in Chapter 1)

If a tumour is small, the prognosis is good, and the smaller the tumour the better the survival. Clinical examination can detect a carcinoma about 1.5 cm in diameter and the hands of an experienced clinician can detect tumours as small as 1.0 cm in diameter.

Screening tests should be simple to perform, cheap, easy, and unambiguous to interpret, and able to identify women with cancer and to exclude those without cancer.

Mammography can detect tumours down to about 0.5 cm and can identify both *in situ* cancers (that have not developed the ability to spread) as well as invasive cancers. However, it is expensive and requires high-technology equipment, special film, dedicated processing, and highly trained radiologists to interpret the films, and it only detects up to 95% of cancers. In addition, not all mammographically suspicious lesions are subsequently confirmed as malignant.

Mammography is currently the best screening tool available for detecting breast cancer, and lowers mortality in randomized trials. Overall these studies indicate an approximate 30% reduction in mortality. Population screening was introduced in the UK in 1988. All women between the ages of 50 and 65 years are invited to have a mammogram at 3-yearly intervals. From 2006 the UK Government has increased the upper age limit to 70 years.

Mammography does, however, have limitations. It is less sensitive in premenopausal woman whose breast tissue is more radiologically 'dense'. The procedure can also be uncomfortable or painful and compliance is less than 100%.

If a woman has a significant abnormality she is asked to come back for further assessment. Further imaging and clinical examination are then performed. If there is a 'composite' shadow that is not seen on subsequent mammography, and if there are no clinical abnormalities, the woman returns to the normal screening round. If there is any doubt, ultrasound-guided fine-needle aspiration cytology (FNAC) and/or core biopsy

are performed. An experienced radiologist, surgeon, and pathologist are present at assessment, and the patient is supported by a breast care nurse. If there is still doubt about the diagnosis, a further biopsy may be needed. If the suspect lesion is impalpable, a marker wire is inserted stereotactically (using imaging techniques to provide a three-dimensional model of the position of the lesion) to guide the surgeon to the suspicious area. An X-ray of the excised tissue is compared with the mammogram to make sure that the suspicious area has been removed. If this procedure is being carried out to establish a diagnosis, care is taken to remove only a small amount of tissue (< 20 g).

Presentation

Clinical and radiological examinations are used to confirm a breast abnormality, the nature of which is determined histologically and cytologically.

- Clinical examination
- Mammography
- Ultrasound (especially for younger women or when mammography is unclear)
- Magnetic resonance imaging (MRI) (occasionally used in younger women, or in the presence of implants, previous surgery, or radiotherapy)
- Fine-needle aspiration
- Core biopsy
- Open biopsy

This approach to diagnosis and staging has > 90% sensitivity and specificity in detecting breast cancer.

Key Facts

Common presentations of breast cancer

- Breast lump
- Breast pain
- Nipple inversion or bloody discharge

The above symptoms account for over 90% of breast cancer presentations.

- Mammographically detected lesion – increasingly common mode of presentation (20%)
- Occasionally rash at nipple (Paget's disease)

Clinical examination

Clinical examination should be carried out by an appropriately trained health professional with a chaperone present.

Women should be examined:

* In a good light to observe for irregularities such as skin dimpling

* Sitting and lying

* With the arm at their side and raised

* With their muscles relaxed and tensed

* Comparison of both breasts is an important assessment, looking for asymmetry

* Examination is incomplete without examining the axillary and supraclavicular lymph nodes

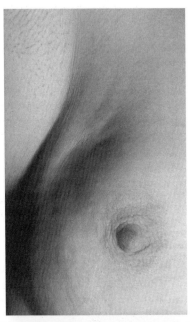

Fig. 10.2 Skin dimpling indicating tethering by carcinoma of the breast.

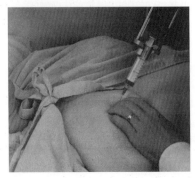

Fig. 10.3 Fine-needle aspiration.

Staging

Routine staging interventions are no longer performed preoperatively in women with early breast cancer.

All patients with proven invasive disease should have the axilla assessed as part of staging. This has been done by axillary clearance as part of primary surgery, but sentinel node biopsy (see page 34) is effective in reducing the number of axillary clearances with less morbidity including pain and lymphoedema.[3]

Women at a higher risk of developing metastatic disease are those with signs or symptoms of metastases, or who have 'high-risk disease' following surgery, e.g. several involved lymph nodes.

The Nottingham Prognostic Index (NPI; see Table 10.4) gives an estimate of prognosis. An on line programme is used to predict potential benefits from adjuvant systemic therapy (adjuvantonline.com).

Stop and Think

The diagnosis of breast cancer has been speeded up in recent years with the goal being to reduce the psychological stress of having to wait for the diagnosis when cancer is possible. However, the one-stop shop approach to diagnosis places particular strains on women attending such a clinically efficient service.

'I was very conscious as I sat there in the waiting room with five other women, that before tea-time statistically at least one of us would be given the news that they had breast cancer.'

TABLE 10.2	Histological grading of invasive breast cancer
Grade I	
Good tubular formation	
Little nuclear pleomorphism	
Few mitotic figures	
Grade II	
A little tubule formation	
Moderate nuclear pleomorphism	
Some mitotic figures	
Grade III	
Little or no tubule formation	
Massive nuclear pleomorphism	
Many mitotic figures	

TABLE 10.3 TNM classification and staging for breast cancer

TNM classification		Stage grouping		
T_{is}	*In situ*	Stage 0	T_{is}	N_0
T_1	≤ 2 cm	Stage I	T_1	N_0
		Stage IIA	T_0	N_1
			T_1	N_1
			T_2	N_0
T_2	> 2–5 cm	Stage IIB	T_2	N_1
T_3	> 5 cm		T_3	N_0
T_4	Chest wall/skin	Stage IIIA	T_0	N_2
			T_1	N_2
			T_2	N_2
			T_3	N_1, N_2
		Stage IIIB	T_4	Any N
			Any T	N_3
pN_0	no nodes involved			
pN_1	1–3 nodes involved			
pN_2	4–9 nodes involved			
pN_3	10+ nodes involved			
M_1	Distant metastases			
		Stage IV	any T and any N	
			M_1	

TABLE 10.4 Nottingham Prognostic Index

NPI = (size of tumour in cm × 0.2) + grade + axillary node score

Axillary node score

0 +ve nodes = 1

1–3 +ve nodes = 2

4 or more +ve nodes = 3

Interpretation

Below 3.5 – prognosis very good

3.6–5.5 – prognosis fair

Over 5.6 – prognosis poor

Oestrogen receptors (ER) and progesterone receptors (PR)

These receptors are present on many breast cancers and are routinely assessed by immunohistochemical techniques. They have prognostic significance in that women whose cancers are ER positive have a better survival than those who are ER negative. In addition, receptor status is a predictive factor, identifying those women who may benefit from endocrine manipulation either as adjuvant therapy or in the metastatic setting.

TABLE 10.5 Management by stage

LCIS	Usually only observed
Non-invasive breast cancer	Excision often followed by post-operative radiotherapy; occasionally mastectomy
	Axillary dissection not indicated
Early breast cancer $T_{1–3}, N_{0–1}$	**Surgery** – either mastectomy or lumpectomy and axillary node dissection
	Loco-regional radiotherapy – indicated for almost all patients after breast conserving surgery and for mastectomy patients at high risk of local relapse (e.g. patients with more than four positive nodes or tumour close to the pectoralis muscle)
	Adjuvant endocrine therapy – indicated for all ER- or PR-positive tumours. Tamoxifen achieves approximately 30% relative reduction in mortality. Aromatase inhibitors are replacing tamoxifen in postmenopausal women because of better outcomes and greater tolerability. The optimal sequence of tamoxifen and aromatase inhibition is still unclear
	Adjuvant chemotherapy – combination chemotherapy reduces recurrence and improves overall survival. Anthracycline-based regimens are more effective than non-anthracycline-based regimens; incorporation of a taxane may further increase efficacy
	Absolute 10-year survival benefit: 7–11% < 50 years; 2–3% > 50 years
	Commonly used regimens include: Doxyrubicin/cyclophosphamide (AC); 5-fluorouracil/epirubicin/cyclophosphamide (FEC); cyclophosphamide/methotrexate/5-fluorouracil (CMF); Docetaxel/Doxyrubicin/cyclophosphamide (TAC)
	In women with Her-2 positive breast cancer, early results of large clinical trials show significant improvements in survival from the addition of trastuzumab. The optimal duration and sequencing of trastuzumab is not yet clear
	The risk:benefit ratio for chemotherapy must be assessed on an individual patient basis
	Neoadjuvant therapy – may allow more women with large tumours to have breast conserving surgery, but appears not to improve survival compared to adjuvant treatment

TABLE 10.5	Management by stage – *continued*
Locally advanced breast cancer	The presence of infiltration of the skin, chest wall, or fixed axillary nodes requires a *neoadjuvant* approach. Younger patients and those with ER/PR-negative disease need chemotherapy
	Elderly patients with ER or PR positive disease may be treated with hormonal therapy alone. In this situation aromatase inhibitors are superior to tamoxifen
Metastatic breast cancer *The aim is palliation* *Usual sites of metastases – lung, liver, bone, and brain. Patients with soft tissue disease may survive for many years*	**Endocrine therapy** – indicated only in those patients with ER or PR positive disease and slowly progressive disease, especially if involving soft tissue rather than visceral sites
	Responses tend to be slower in onset (3–6 months) than with chemotherapy but also tend to be more durable
	Expected response rates of 40–60% to first-line hormonal therapy
	Disease that responds to endocrine therapy and then progresses has a 25% response rate with second-line endocrine treatment
	Response to a third hormonal agent is 10–15%
	Chemotherapy – chemotherapy is indicated in situations where a high response rate and rapid response are required and in those with ER/PR-negative tumours or who have not responded to endocrine therapy
	Anthracyclines, either as single agents or in combination, are used in patients not exposed to them in the adjuvant setting. First-line response rates are over 40–60%. After anthracyclines, taxanes (paclitaxel or docetaxel) have active response rates similar to those above, again as single agents or in combination. Other cytotoxics with significant activity include oral capecitabine, vinorelbine, and liposomal doxorubicin
	In patients with HER-2 overexpression, the addition of trastuzumab (Herceptin®) increases response rate and prolongs survival. Herceptin® may also be used as a single agent
	Radiotherapy – useful for palliation of painful bone metastases or of soft tissue metastases causing pressure effects as well as brain metastases and spinal cord compression
	Bisphosphonates – useful in the treatment of hypercalcaemia and bone pain even when bone metastases cannot be detected
	In patients with bone metastases they reduce bone pain and skeletal events related to malignancy and the incidence of hypercalcaemia

HER-2 receptors

About 20% of breast cancers overexpress the Her-2 cell surface receptor. This is associated with a poor prognosis, but has become a therapeutic target.

Trastuzumab is a monoclonal antibody that blocks the HER-2 receptor. 2005 trials show survival benefit in the early adjuvant setting in Her-2 positive patients for Herceptin.

In advanced disease trastuzumab can shrink Her-2 +ve tumours when used either as a single agent or in combination with chemotherapy, and significantly prolongs survival.

Management

Management of breast cancer in women over 70

The elderly woman should be treated in the same way as her 'younger sister' taking into account her general health. A wide local excision or a mastectomy can be performed under local anaesthesia, and older women often tolerate radiotherapy well.

If she is fit for general anaesthesia then the axilla should be cleared. All elderly patients should be considered for adjuvant treatment. If their cancers are ER/PR positive they should be offered tamoxifen or an aromatase inhibitor. Those with especially high-risk disease, or ER/PR negative disease, should be considered for adjuvant chemotherapy if they are otherwise fit. There is a small group of very elderly or unfit patients who cannot be treated surgically. For these women,

---

Key Facts

Surgery in breast cancer

- Historically, surgery invariably involved a disfiguring mastectomy

- It is now clear that >50% cancers can be treated 'conservatively' by excision of the tumour and a rim of normal tissue (>0.5 cm) followed by radiotherapy

- Breast conservation surgery is not always an option, e.g. large tumours in women with small breasts, where conservation may be technically impossible or result in an unacceptable cosmetic effect

- Survival outcomes comparing mastectomy and conservation are equivalent provided appropriate adjuvant therapy is given

- Where both mastectomy and conservation are options, 'patient choice', with the woman expressing her preference, is offered

endocrine therapy may be given as a sole treatment; in the majority it will hold the disease in check for at least 2 years if their cancer is ER/PR positive.

Breast cancer and pregnancy

◆ Two breast cancers occur in every 10,000 women who are pregnant

◆ These unfortunate women should have surgery as soon as possible, but preferably after the first trimester and with consideration of the risks of inducing labour in later pregnancy

◆ Chemotherapy can be used in the mid and last trimesters

Male breast cancer

◆ Carcinoma of the male breast is uncommon, accounting for less than 1% of all breast cancers

◆ The prognosis and the response to treatment are remarkably similar between the sexes

◆ The pathology of male breast cancer is similar to that in women

◆ *The vast majority are infiltrating ductal carcinoma*

◆ Primary treatment is with mastectomy and axillary node clearance

◆ Radiotherapy is given postoperatively because of the proximity of the pectoralis muscle

◆ As a high percentage of male breast carcinomas are ER-positive they often benefit from hormone treatment. Those with ER/PR-negative disease or with high-risk cancers are offered adjuvant chemotherapy

◆ Survival is good for men whose disease is node negative, 80% surviving 5 years, but only 46% of men with node-positive tumours are alive at 5 years

Paget's disease of the nipple

Paget's disease presents as a rash caused by invasion of cancer cells (Paget's cells) into the epidermis of the nipple and areola. It is distinguished from eczema which involves the areola alone.

If Paget's disease is diagnosed histologically, treatment is a total mastectomy; excision of the nipple alone gives a poor cosmetic result. Adjuvant treatment would depend on ER, and menopausal status.

Paget's disease of the nipple:

◆ Can only definitely be diagnosed by a full thickness skin biopsy

◆ Is only associated with 1–2% of breast cancers

◆ Occurs on the nipple and areola whereas eczema is confined to the areola

◆ A mammogram may pinpoint the underlying cancer

◆ The only effective treatment is a total mastectomy

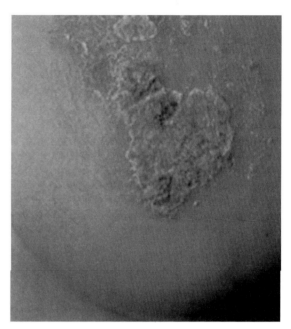

Fig. 10.4 Paget's disease of the nipple.

Stop and Think

Reconstruction after mastectomy

The majority of women first want to be sure that the cancer is removed, and only secondly are concerned with their shape. However, there are those to whom body shape is as important as eradicating the cancer, and who request an operation to reconstruct the breast. The choice of operation for an individual patient includes the use of implants or reconstruction using muscle flaps. The operation can be done at the initial cancer surgery or delayed until later.

The psychological effects of breast surgery can be profound with sexuality and body image issues having the potential to put a strain on even the most robust of relationships.

Support from specialist nurses who are experienced in such matters may reduce the associated morbidity.

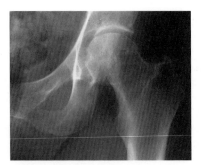

Fig. 10.5 Pathological fracture of neck of femur.

Common problems associated with progressive disease

When a patient's breast cancer progresses, she is staged clinically and radiologically to assess the extent of the disease and her symptoms are also assessed. Treatment options will be one or more of: (1) a change in systemic therapy (chemotherapy, endocrine therapy or trastuzumab), especially for widespread disease; (2) local treatment (radiotherapy or surgery) when one disease site causes particular concern, for example, a pleural effusion; and (3) symptomatic measures (analgesics, bisphosphonates)

- **Bone pain** as a result of bone metastases may require radiotherapy, bisphosphonates, or change of systemic therapy. Bisphonates can also inhibit metastatic progression in bone. Prophylactic surgery may be indicated where there is a risk of fracture

- **Pathological fracture**s may occur without obvious trauma and need surgical fixation followed by radiotherapy

- **Spinal cord compression** requires prompt diagnosis, high-dose oral steroids, and urgent referral to the oncologist. The steroids should be continued at a high dose until a definitive plan has been made. The diagnosis is confirmed by MRI, and surgery or radiotherapy is instigated urgently

- **Neuropathic pain** can be a particular problem especially if there has been spread into the brachial plexus. Sometimes it is difficult to differentiate between recurrence or the effects of radiotherapy

- **Liver metastases** are common and may require steroids or non-steroidal anti-inflammatory drugs to reduce the pain of liver capsule stretch in addition to systemic therapy

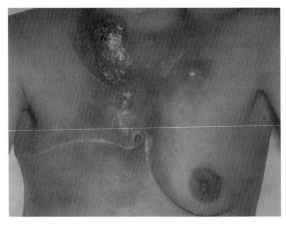

Fig. 10.6 Local recurrence photograph courtesy of Dr Caroline Lucas, Princess Alice Hospital, Esher.

- **Hypercalcaemia** may occur. In symptomatic cases treatment should be considered urgently with intravenous hydration and bisphosphonates. Oral bisphosphonates may have a place in more chronic situations.

- **Local recurrence** can lead to the breakdown of skin over the chest wall or axilla. Radiotherapy may be helpful if not previously administered to the affected area, otherwise a change in systemic therapy will be considered. Meticulous skin care and management are necessary to reduce the distressing effects of odour and discharge

- **Lymphoedema** (swelling of the arm) can develop at any point in the course of the disease. In the past this was often severe, caused by a combination of radiotherapy and surgery to the axilla. This is less common with current approaches to the axilla. Early referral to a lymphoedema specialist provides the best chance of minimizing the morbidity and distress caused. Management includes good skin care, avoiding additional trauma to the affected arm (including taking blood tests and blood pressure measurements), and appropriately fitting compression garments

- **Lung and pleural spread** are common causes of breathlessness and cough. These symptoms need to be investigated thoroughly. Drainage of a pleural effusion may be a useful symptomatic procedure. Pleurodesis should be considered, especially if the patient does not have other life-threatening metastatic disease. A change in systemic therapy, usually chemotherapy, should be considered

◆ **Psychosocial problems**. Some of these patients will be mothers with young children for whom the trauma of disease is worsened by fears for their children. A multidisciplinary supportive approach at a pace dictated by the patient can help to reduce some of the distress for the patient and her family. A major factor can be a pre-death bereavement state through which a woman may grieve for her physical, emotional, professional, maternal, and sexual identities and for social losses. There is accumulating evidence that psychosocial support influences adjustment to cancer, and clinical observations in various settings suggest that factors ranging from pain control to mortality can be altered by such support. This support can be offered by medical personnel, specialist breast care nurses, psychologists, support groups, volunteers, and the families of patients

---

CASE HISTORY

Test Yourself

CAN: Post-menopausal woman with breast carcinoma

Mrs CAN was aged 62 when she went to the NHS Breast Screening Centre for a mammogram, and as the mammogram showed an abnormality she was asked to attend an assessment clinic. She had not noticed any abnormality in her breast, and, even after the invitation to attend the assessment clinic arrived, she still could not find any abnormality. She was extremely anxious when she received the recall letter.

Mrs CAN has four children. The oldest one was born when she was aged 30, and she had her first period when she was aged 11. When she was aged 52 she experienced the menopause, and was put on HRT. She stopped this therapy 2 years ago. Her mother had breast cancer, treated with a mastectomy, when she was aged 58. Her mother subsequently died of a heart attack aged 81.

1. What factors contribute to Mrs CAN's risk of developing breast cancer?

At the assessment clinic the doctor could not palpate any abnormality, but repeat mammograms showed a spiculated lesion behind the left nipple which was 0.5 cm in diameter. FNAC under ultrasound control confirmed that this lesion was malignant.

Diagnostic summary

◆ Screening mammogram: suspicious

◆ Assessment mammography: malignant

◆ Ultrasound-guided FNAC: malignant

◆ Clinical examination: no lesion discovered

Mrs CAN was advised that wide local excision would give a poor cosmetic result as the lesion was behind the nipple, so she chose a mastectomy. She was very distressed by the diagnosis and needed the support of the breast care nurse at the assessment clinic, and prior to admission. Six days after the triple assessment, she had a left mastectomy and axillary node clearance.

The level I, II, and III nodes were cleared from the axilla. There was a suction drain behind the mastectomy wound and another suction drain in the axilla when she returned from theatre. These were removed at 48 hours and 72 hours, respectively, and then Mrs CAN went home.

A 0.6-cm tumour was found behind the left nipple. The margins of excision were clear of tumour. Histologically, the tumour showed much tubule formation, the nuclei were very uniform and small in size, and there were only two mitotic figures per high-power field. This is a grade II tumour (1,2,1). There were no metastases in the 18 lymph nodes recovered from the axilla. ERs were positive, as were PRs.

Pathological summary

◆ Size of the tumour: 0.6 cm

◆ Grade of the tumour: II (1,2,1)

◆ Axillary nodes: level I, 0/12, level II, 0/4, level III, 0/2

◆ ER positive

◆ PR positive

The NBI was 3.12 and the prognosis for Mrs CAN is therefore good.

2. What treatments would you now recommend and why?

Test Yourself

ROD: Pre-menopausal woman with breast carcinoma

Mrs ROD was aged 42 when she found a lump in her right breast. She was a married woman with three children. Her first baby was born when she was aged 23 and she had her first period when she was aged 13. She has no family history of breast cancer, and took the oral contraceptive pill from the age of 30 to the age of 40. Her menstrual cycle was regular and normal.

1. What factors contribute to Mrs ROD's risk of developing breast cancer?

She went to her GP who referred her to the breast clinic. He confirmed that she had a 2×2-cm lump in the upper outer quadrant of the right breast. There was no skin attachment, and no attachment to deep fascia. No glands could be palpated in the axilla or supraclavicular fossa. There was no liver enlargement, no abnormal signs in the chest, and no tenderness over bone prominences. A mammogram showed that this mass had the characteristics of malignancy, and FNAC, under ultrasound control to ensure the needle was in the lesion, showed malignant cells.

Diagnostic summary

◆ Aged 42 (premenopausal)

◆ Palpable lump 2×2 cm

◆ Mammogram – carcinoma

◆ Ultrasound – malignant

◆ FNAC – malignant

After discussion with the surgeon and the breast care nurse, Mrs ROD chose to have a partial mastectomy and axillary node clearance. This was performed 1 week after her attendance at the breast clinic, and she was in hospital for 3 days. An axillary drain was left in place after the operation, and this was removed

after 48 hours. She was mobile and helping to hand out tea in the ward on the morning of discharge. The breast care nurses had taught her exercises to prevent shoulder stiffness, and she felt very well.

Pathology revealed a 1.8-cm tumour had been excised, and the margins of excision were 5 mm distant from the nearest tumour edge. There were 12 lymph nodes found in level 1, of which four contained metastases, and there were three lymph nodes found in level 2, of which one contained a metastasis. Histologically, the tumour did not show any tubule formation, the nuclei were very pleomorphic, and there were 26 mitoses per high-power field. ERs and PRs were negative.

Pathological summary

◆ Size 1.8 cm

◆ Grade III (3,3,3)

◆ Axillary nodes: level I, 4/12, level II, 1/4, level III, 0/2, total 5/18

◆ ERs negative

◆ PRs negative

2. What treatment would you recommend and why?

The NPI was 6.36 so Mrs ROD is at high risk of recurrence. After discussion at a multidisciplinary team meeting Mrs ROD was referred to the oncologists, who gave her radiotherapy and chemotherapy.

The radiotherapy was given to the breast in 25 fractions over 5 weeks, and the chemotherapy was doxyrubicin and cyclophosphamide, given every 3 weeks for four courses. Unfortunately, her hair fell out, but had regrown by the end of the treatment.

She remained well until 1 year and 6 months after her treatment when she began to have nausea. She went to see her GP, who noted that she was jaundiced, and sent her urgently to the oncologist. She was noted to have liver secondaries and started a course of Taxotere®, but did not improve. She went downhill rapidly, and died peacefully 1 year and 9 months after the initial diagnosis.

Chapter summary

- Accounts for 20% of all cancers
- Lifetime risk in women is 1 in 9
- Factors which increase the risk of breast cancer include increasing age, a family history of breast cancer, nulliparity, and use of hormone replacement therapy (HRT)
- 5–10% of breast cancers are believed to be hereditary

Screening

- Mammography is expensive but effective.
- It requires high-technology equipment, special film, and dedicated processing, and highly trained radiologists to interpret the films, and it detects only 90–95% of cancers

Breast cancer is diagnosed by

- Mammogram
- Ultrasound is now complementary to mammography
- Fine-needle aspiration cytology (FNAC) or core biopsy
- MRI occasionally – for young women, or in the presence of implants, previous surgery, or radiotherapy

Prognostic factors include

- Axillary node involvement – most important prognostic criterion
- Tumour size
- Tumour grade
- Oestrogen receptor (ER)/progesterone receptor (PR) status

Management

- Non-invasive breast cancer ductal carcinoma *in situ* (DCIS) – usually local excision and post-operative radiotherapy
- Early breast cancer
  - Surgery (wide local excision or mastectomy)
  - Locoregional radiotherapy
  - Adjuvant endocrine therapy
  - Adjuvant chemotherapy (+/– Herceptin)
- Locally advanced breast cancer
  - Neoadjuvant systems treatment
  - Local treatment with surgery/radiotherapy
- Metastatic breast cancer
  - Endocrine therapy
  - Chemotherapy (+/– Herceptin)
  - Radiotherapy
  - Bisphosphonates
- The older woman should be treated in the same way as her 'younger sister'
- There is a small group of very elderly or unfit patients who cannot be treated surgically who may benefit from endocrine therapy

References

1. http://info.cancerresearchuk.org/cancerstats/types/breast/incidence/
2. http://info.cancerresearchuk.org/cancerstats/types/breast/mortality/
3. Clarke D, *et al.* The learning curve in sentinel node biopsy: the ALMANAC experience. *Annals of Surgical Oucology* 2004, **11**(3 suppl), 211S–215S.

Case studies and multiple choice questions at www.oxfordtextbooks.co.uk/orc/watson/

Patients with common gynaecological cancers

Ovarian carcinoma

Incidence and mortality

In 2001 6,883 women were diagnosed with ovarian cancer in the UK.[1]

In 2003 4,617 women died from ovarian cancer in the UK.[2]

Background

◆ Fifth commonest cancer in women

◆ Commonest gynaecological cancer in the UK

◆ Risk is reduced by factors that reduce the number of ovulatory cycles, e.g. pregnancy, prolonged use of oral contraceptive pill

◆ Approximately 5% are familial

◆ Median age at diagnosis 66 years

◆ > 90% of tumours are epithelial in origin

  • Serous adenocarcinoma 40–50%

  • Endometrioid 15–30%

  • Mucinoid and clear cell 10–15% each

◆ Spread is predominantly to other organs in the pelvic cavity and is often associated with ascites. Later spread may be to the chest and liver parenchyma

◆ 5-year survival less than 25%

Presentation

Ovarian cancer spreads mainly intraperitoneally and may often remain 'silent' until the disease is advanced; 80% of patients, therefore, present with disease which has spread beyond the pelvis.

Key Facts

Genetics and ovarian cancer

- 5% of women have a family history of two or more relatives with ovarian cancer

- 5% have one relative with ovarian cancer and a history of another family member with either breast, endometrial or bowel cancer

- Two genes, *BRAC1* and *BRAC2*, have been implicated

Future Possibilities

Screening and ovarian cancer

- Currently under study for women perceived to be at high risk

- Ultrasound has high sensitivity (98%)

- Coupled with colour flow Doppler studies, ultrasound also has a high specificity (97%)

- Both these methods are labour intensive

- Serum CA-125 has a sensitivity of 70–80% and a specificity of 98%

- As yet no investigations are deemed suitable for mass screening but trials are ongoing

Common presenting symptoms include:

- Abdominal distension

- Abdominal pain

- Altered bowel habit

- Weight loss

Examination

Such symptoms should trigger clinical suspicion and prompt examination to distinguish between 'fat, flatus, fluid, and tumour' on abdominal, vaginal, and rectal assessment.

If cancer is suspected, ultrasound examination and CA-125 estimation should be undertaken.

Diagnosis and staging

Pre-operatively a diagnosis of ovarian cancer may be suspected by a raised CA-125 (elevated in approximately 85% of patients with stage III/IV disease) and the presence of a pelvic mass or ascites on computerized tomography scan.

TABLE 11.1	International Federation of Gynaecology and Obstetrics (FIGO) classification of the stages of ovarian carcinoma
Stage I	Growth limited to the ovaries
Stage Ia	Growth limited to one ovary; no ascites present containing malignant cells. No tumour on the external surface; capsule intact
Stage Ib	Growth limited to both ovaries; no ascites present containing malignant cells; no tumour on the external surfaces; capsules intact
Stage Ic	Tumour stage Ia or Ib but with tumour on surface of one or both ovaries; or with capsule ruptured; or with ascites present containing malignant cells or with positive peritoneal washings
Stage II	Growth involving one or both ovaries with pelvic extension
Stage IIa	Extension and/or metastases to the uterus and/or tubes
Stage IIb	Extension to other pelvic tissues
Stage IIc	Tumour stage IIa or IIb but with tumour on surface of one or both ovaries; or with capsule(s) ruptured; or with ascites present containing malignant cells or with positive peritoneal washings
Stage III	Tumour involving one or both ovaries with peritoneal implants outside the pelvis and/or positive retroperitoneal or inguinal nodes; superficial liver metastases. Tumour is limited to the true pelvis but with histologically proven malignant extension to small bowel or omentum
Stage IIIa	Tumour grossly limited to the true pelvis with negative nodes but with histologically confirmed microscopic seeding of abdominal peritoneal surfaces
Stage IIIb	Tumour of one or both ovaries with histologically confirmed implants of abdominal peritoneal surfaces, none exceeding 2 cm in diameter; nodes are negative
Stage IIIc	Abdominal implants greater than 2 cm in diameter and/or positive retroperitoneal or inguinal nodes
Stage IV	Growth involving one or both ovaries with distant metastases. If pleural effusion is present there must be positive cytology to allot a case to stage IV. Parenchymal liver metastases

TABLE 11.2	Prognosis summary for ovarian carcinoma	
Stage	Description	Five-year survival
Stage I	Confined to ovaries but with no pelvic extension	75%
Stage II	Tumour with pelvic extension	45%
Stage III	Tumour with peritoneal spread outside the pelvis, or involving small bowel; retroperitoneal or inguinal nodes	20%
Stage IV	Distant metastases	<5%

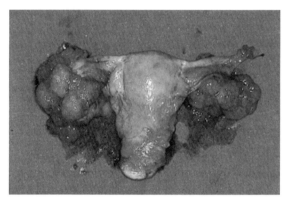

Fig. 11.1 Bilateral ovarian cancers which have breached the capsule of the ovary.

Confirmation of the diagnosis requires histological examination.

In the absence of overt metastatic disease, optimal staging and management require total abdominal hysterectomy (TAH), bilateral salpingo-oophorectomy (BSO), omentectomy, lymph node sampling, and multiple peritoneal biopsies.

Management

Surgery

The main treatment aim of ovarian cancer is to remove as much tumour as possible surgically and then follow with chemotherapy. The bulk of tumour pre-operatively and the amount left post-operatively both impact on ultimate survival. Radical surgery has an important role in treatment and retrospective studies demonstrate significantly improved survival in patients whose disease has been optimally debulked (i.e. no tumour remaining measuring > 1 cm in diameter). Trials of laparoscopic surgery are ongoing.

Stop and Think

How do you consent a patient for surgery when you are unsure how much surgery will be required?

Where optimal debulking is not initially possible there may be a survival benefit from performing debulking surgery after three cycles of chemotherapy – so-called interval debulking.

Exceptions

Important exceptions to the above management plan are the rare germ cell tumours and teratomas which usually respond very well to chemotherapy as primary treatment, which may produce a cure with preserved fertility.

First-line chemotherapy

A platinum/taxane combination is considered by most oncologists to be the optimum treatment for epithelial ovarian cancer, the most commonly used combination being carboplatin and paclitaxel.

Response rates are approximately 70–80%, and median survival is 2–3 years with such treatment.

Although the introduction of paclitaxel has improved the median survival in this disease, the majority of patients develop progressive disease and 5-year survival is still less than 25%.

Treatment at relapse

The majority of patients who relapse after first-line therapy are incurable. Secondary surgical debulking may be useful in selected patients but its value is uncertain. The choice of further chemotherapy depends on the length of interval between completion of previous chemotherapy and relapse. The response rate depends on the 'time out' from treatment, ranging from very low for < 6 months to 60% for > 2 years.

◆ Patients relapsing more than 6 months after completion of platinum-based therapy may respond to further platinum-based chemotherapy and should generally be rechallenged with a platinum agent

◆ Patients relapsing less than 6 months after completion of platinum-based chemotherapy are unlikely to respond to further platinum-based therapy. Fit patients should be considered for liposomal doxorubicin (Caelyx®) or topotecan

CASE HISTORY

'I seem to be losing weight yet my skirt size is getting bigger'

Presentation

Mrs JM is 57 and lives with her husband; they have one grown-up daughter. She has lost her appetite and experienced dyspepsia for the past 5 months. She has also noticed increasing constipation and occasional tenesmus. Her GP has suspected diverticular disease and given dietary advice; he arranged a barium enema, which was normal. Mrs JM developed severe pain in her abdomen and was admitted to hospital with suspected appendicitis. After admission an ultrasound examination of her abdomen confirmed the presence of cystic and solid mass, 12 cm in diameter, arising out of the pelvis with associated free fluid.

Examination

On palpation, the abdomen was slightly distended with a doughy feel. There was a shifting dullness and a fluid thrill. There was the impression of a mass arising out of the right side of the pelvis, which was moderately tender, firm, and irregular, and not mobile.

Speculum examination was normal; vaginal and rectal examination revealed a fixed pelvic mass on the right side of the pelvis almost filling the pelvis and attached to the uterus.

Management

Chest X-ray, full blood count, urea & electrolytes, liver function tests, CA-125, and CT scans were arranged.

The patient and her husband were counselled regarding the probable diagnosis of ovarian cancer and advised as to the surgery required. They agreed to this and surgery was scheduled as soon as possible because the patient was in pain.

At laparotomy, after draining 2500 ml of ascitic fluid, a 12-cm ovarian tumour of the right ovary was found, which was fixed to the side of the pelvis and invading the uterus; a loop of terminal ileum was densely adherent to the top of the tumour as was the serosa of the anterior wall of the rectum. The left ovary was normal. There were several studs of tumour 1–2 cm in the omentum and a couple of tiny nodules 3 mm in diameter over the peritoneum, the bladder, and right paracolic gutter. The tumour was staged as FIGO IIIb.

A total hysterectomy, bilateral salpingo-oophorectomy and omentectomy were performed. All other visible tumour nodules were excised including some residual tumour of the serosa of the rectum. The tumour was invading deeply into the wall of the ileum and this part was resected with primary anastomosis of the bowel.

At the end of the operation there was no residual tumour to be seen.

Mrs JM made a satisfactory postoperative recovery and was referred for chemotherapy.

Six cycles of cisplatin and paclitaxel were administered on a 4-weekly basis. At the end of treatment, Mrs JM was feeling well, her serum CA-125 had fallen from 1395 U/ml pre-operatively to 24 U/ml and arrangements were made for 3-monthly follow-up at the joint oncology clinic.

Eventually all patients who relapse following primary chemotherapy will develop chemotherapy-resistant disease. The majority of these patients will have symptoms related to intra-abdominal disease including abdominal pain and bowel obstruction. Management of these symptoms can be very challenging and requires a multidisciplinary approach with involvement of palliative care physicians, surgeons, and oncologists.

 Case studies and multiple choice questions at www.oxfordtextbooks.co.uk/orc/watson/

Endometrial cancer

Incidence and mortality

In 2001 5,646 women were diagnosed with endometrial cancer in the UK.[3]

In 2003 1,059 women died from endometrial cancer in the UK.[4]

Background

◆ Endometrial cancer incidence is gradually increasing and has now overtaken cervical cancer in incidence in the UK and USA

◆ Endometrial cancer is almost always a disease of post-menopausal woman (age range 55–70 years) and is very rare before the age of 40

◆ Endometrial cancer is closely associated with obesity, low parity, and late menopause; it is also associated with hypertension and diabetes

◆ In the 1970s in the USA there was a documented rise in the incidence of endometrial cancer, which was linked with the administration of unopposed oestrogens to post-menopausal women to control climacteric symptoms

- There is also clinical evidence of an association between endometrial carcinoma and high circulating oestrogen levels, e.g. polycystic ovarian syndrome and oestrogen-producing tumours, where chronic anovulation with raised oestrogen production causes endometrial abnormalities

- Concern has been raised about the long-term administration of tamoxifen to women with breast cancer. Although tamoxifen is an anti-oestrogen and blocks oestrogen receptors in breast tissue, it is also a partial agonist and has some stimulatory activity. It is now clear that long-term use increases the risk of endometrial cancer

Pathology

- Approximately 60–70% of endometrial malignancies are adenocarcinoma

- Other tumours described are adenoacanthoma, adenosquamous, clear cell and mixed Müllerian (carcinosarcomas)

- The microscopic appearances of adenocarcinoma range from very well-differentiated tumours (50%) indistinguishable from atypical hyperplasia through moderate differentiation (30%) to very poorly differentiated or anaplastic lesions, which have lost virtually all glandular patterns (20%)

- Because of the influence of differentiation on management, lesions should be labelled according to the worst grade of differentiation found

Presentation

Classically, endometrial tumours present with post-menopausal bleeding and all women experiencing abnormal bleeding in the peri-menopausal years or afterwards must have investigations to exclude malignancy.

Diagnosis

Patients with post-menopausal bleeding should have a vaginal ultrasound to define endometrial thickness (normally < 4 mm after the menopause) and an endometrial sample taken for histological examination. This latter investigation is the subject of controversy as some investigators question its accuracy. The main diagnostic investigation is hysteroscopy and biopsy, which may be performed under local or general anaes-

TABLE 11.3	Staging of endometrial cancer
Stage Ia	Tumour limited to endometrium
Stage Ib	Invasion to less than half the myometrium
Stage Ic	Invasion to more than half the myometrium
Stage IIa	Endocervical glandular involvement only
Stage IIb	Cervical serosal invasion
Stage IIIa	Tumour invades serosa and/or adnexae
Stage IIIb	Vaginal metastases
Stage IIIc	Metastases to pelvic and/or para-aortic lymph nodes
Stage IVa	Tumour invasion of bladder and/or bowel mucosa
Stage IVb	Distant metastases, including intra-abdominal and/or inguinal lymph nodes

thetic. This has the advantage of identifying the site of the lesion and obtaining a directed biopsy.

Investigation

Hysteroscopy will determine the site of the lesion, i.e. fundal or involving the cervical os.

It will also enable a directly viewed representative biopsy to be performed, an estimation of uterine cavity size, and the presence or absence of other uterine pathology.

Bi-manual pelvic examination should also be carried out to assess for adnexal pathology (there is a 5% incidence of concomitant tumours of the ovary).

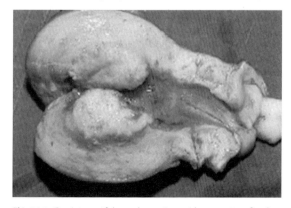

Fig. 11.2 Carcinoma of the endometrium with tumour confined to the inner half of the myometrium.

Once the diagnosis is confirmed, a magnetic resonance imaging (MRI) or spiral CT scan should be carried out. The former is useful in determining the depth of tumour invasion pre-operatively and also assessing lymphadenopathy in the pelvis, whilst the latter is more useful in visualizing abdominal lymph nodes and chest metastases (a chest X-ray would probably suffice, however, in the majority of cases).

Treatment

- Standard treatment for the past 25 years for endometrial cancer has been TAH and BSO followed by radiotherapy if adverse prognostic factors are identified at histology, i.e. cervical extension, poorly differentiated histology, and deep myometrial involvement

- With improved pre-operative assessment, most of this information should be known before surgery and patients more carefully selected for treatment. Patients with early stage I disease without deep myometrial involvement and well-differentiated tumours may be treated by TAH and BSO alone

- More advanced stage I and stage II tumours need either adjuvant radiotherapy after surgery or should be treated with radical hysterectomy and lymph node sampling with post-operative radiotherapy given for stage Ic–II disease

- More advanced disease should be treated with radiotherapy, both external beam and intracavitary, followed by surgery if residual central disease persists

- Conventional chemotherapy gives very poor cure rates in this disease and is rarely used outside clinical trials except occasionally for palliation

---

CASE HISTORY

Test Yourself

SN: 'My periods have returned after 10 years – I did not think this was possible'

History

Mrs SN was a 65-year-old married woman who had two children. She weighed 97 kg was taking a β-blocker for moderate hypertension and was a non-insulin-dependent diabetic controlled by diet alone. She had a delayed menopause but never took hormone replacement therapy. She noticed blood on her pants after attending the funeral of her sister who had died from metastatic breast cancer after several years' treatment and thought that it was due to shock. The bleeding persisted and became like a period lasting 6 days.

1. What risk factors did Mrs SN have for developing endometrial carcinoma?

Examination

Mrs SN was markedly obese and abdominal palpation was unrewarding.

Speculum examination showed a cystocele and normal cervix. There was blood coming through the cervical os.

Management

Mrs SN was referred to her local gynaecologist who performed vaginal ultrasound, finding an enlarged uterus and thickened endometrium.

An outpatient endometrial sample revealed 'cheesy' endometrium, which, on histological examination, showed adenocarcinoma cells.

A hysteroscopy under anaesthetic showed an enlarged uterine wall (9 mm) and a polypoid, pale lesion arising from the uterine fundus. A biopsy was performed, which confirmed the diagnosis of a poorly differentiated adenocarcinoma.

A chest X-ray and MRI scan were organized. The latter showed that the tumour had not invaded more than a third of the way into the myometrium; no lymphadenopathy was detected.

2. How would you stage Mrs SN's tumour?
The patient was referred to the gynaecological cancer centre for surgery. An extended hysterectomy, bilateral salpingo-oophorectomy, and pelvic and para-aortic node dissection were performed.

Histology revealed that the tumour had poorly differentiated elements, invasion was confined to the inner third of the myometrium, and all the lymph nodes were normal.

After discussion it was decided not to give adjuvant treatment as the tumour did not show evidence of spread and 5 years later Mrs SN remained well and disease free.

◆ Tumours may show sensitivity to progestogens, particularly those that are well differentiated. Use of progestogens is generally limited to treatment of advanced or recurrent disease

Prognosis

◆ Because endometrial carcinoma tends to present at an early stage with post-menopausal bleeding and is commonly a stage I, well-differentiated lesion, the overall outcome is 70% 5-year disease-free survival

◆ Poor differentiation, deep myometrial invasion, and lymph node metastases all confer an adverse prognosis and it is this group that should be identified pre-operatively if possible and selected for a more aggressive treatment strategy

◆ One other group, in which a poor outcome may be expected, are those patients with carcinosarcoma. These tumours behave in a very aggressive manner and there may be micrometastases in the lung or brain by the time of diagnosis, making effective therapy almost impossible. Chemotherapy with doxorubicin and platinum or ifosfamide may be appropriate

Carcinoma of the cervix

Incidence and mortality

In 2001 2,942 women were diagnosed with cervical cancer in the UK.[5]

In 2003 1,098 women died from cervical cancer in the UK.[6]

Background

◆ Predominantly affects women over 45 years

◆ Second commonest cancer in women worldwide

◆ Incidence is decreasing in countries with a well-developed screening programme

◆ Early intercourse, multiple partners, and male promiscuity indicate the likelihood of a sexually transmitted oncogenic factor

◆ Strongly associated with human papillomavirus (HPV) type 16 (and also, but less strongly, with HPV 18 and 31)

◆ 30–40% of patients with untreated cervical intraepithelial neoplasia progress to invasive squamous cell carcinoma with a latent period of 10–20 years

◆ Commonest female cancer in South East Asia, Africa, and South America

---

Test Yourself

Cervical screening

In the UK in 1988 a national screening programme was initiated which aimed to screen 80% of eligible women aged between 25 and 65 years within 5 years. This was achieved.

The screening method relies on a well-taken sample of cervical cells from the squamous–columnar junction, prompt fixation, good pathology analysis, and excellent record keeping and patient tracking.

Worryingly 50% of cervical cancers in 1995/6 arose in women who had not had a smear within the previous 5 years. Many of these women were in high-risk categories.

Why do you think this happened?

◆ In the UK, incidence and mortality have fallen by approximately 40% since the 1970s

Pathology

◆ 75% of cervical cancers are squamous in origin, 15% are adenocarcinoma, and the rest are clear cell, adenosquamous, and undifferentiated tumours

◆ Squamous tumours arise from the cervical–columnar junction as a result of malignant transformation of metaplastic cells

◆ Tumour invasion is by direct spread into surrounding tissues, into the vaginal epithelium, and the para-cervical tissues towards the pelvic wall

◆ Lymphatic spread to the deep pelvic lymph nodes and external iliac, common iliac, para-aortic chains

◆ Blood spread is less common

Colposcopy is used to examine, treat, and follow-up patients with pre-malignant disease which has usually been detected at cervical screening.

Presentation

◆ Unless detected at screening, often asymptomatic until disease is advanced

◆ Post-coital bleeding

◆ Inter-menstrual bleeding

◆ Examination by speculum may reveal a polypoid mass or an ulcerated lesion in advanced disease

◆ On bimanual examination the cervix may feel hard and mobility will be reduced in advanced disease

Stop and Think

Sexuality and gynaecological surgery

Gynaecological surgery can have a profound effect on a patient's sexuality which can be increased by fear that resuming intercourse may cause pain or damage. Partners may also be fearful that resumption of sexual activity will be a source of distress. Often couples will be shy about raising such matters in a busy outpatients' clinic. Professionals have frequently avoided the subject for fear of causing embarrassment compounding the considerable stress and strain on relationships. Raising the matter routinely, access to written information, opportunities to discuss matters with a nurse specialist or counsellor, and clear explicit advice will reduce much of this important aspect of post-surgical morbidity.

Future Possibilities

Immunization against cervical cancer

Trials of a vaccine against HPV have been successfully completed. These trials have increased the likelihood that within a few years there will be a national immunization programme in the UK which will have a dramatic impact on the incidence of cervical cancer.

Management

Management depends largely on disease stage and the availability of treatments.

In countries where good surgical facilities exist, patients with early-stage disease are offered the choice of radiotherapy or radical surgery (I–IIa) with an outcome of 75% 5-year survival.

Patients with stage Ia disease may be treated with simple hysterectomy, or a conization procedure if they wish to preserve their fertility.

For stage Ib or IIa disease, radical hysterectomy appears equivalent to radical pelvic radiotherapy.

For patients with stage IIb to IVa disease, recent evidence suggests that combined radical pelvic radiotherapy with platinum-based chemotherapy gives the best results.

Chemoradiotherapy may also be indicated for patients with Stage Ib and IIa disease with adverse prognostic factors such as those with bulky tumours.

For patients with Stage IVb disease, pelvic radiotherapy may be useful in palliating troublesome pelvic symptoms. Cervical cancer is only moderately chemosensitive, with responses to single agents of around 20–30%. Agents with some activity in this disease include cisplatin, ifosfamide, and paclitaxel.

Staging

TABLE 11.4	**FIGO staging system**

Ia	Micro-invasive disease (max. depth 5 mm, max. width 7 mm)
Ib	Clinical disease confined to the cervix
IIa	Disease involves upper two-thirds of vagina but not parametrium
IIb	Disease involves parametrium but not pelvic wall
IIIa	Disease involves lower one-third of vagina
IIIb	Disease extends to pelvic side wall
IVa	Spread of tumour to adjacent organs
IVb	Spread to distant organs

MRI plays an increasingly important role in the pre-operative staging of these tumours.

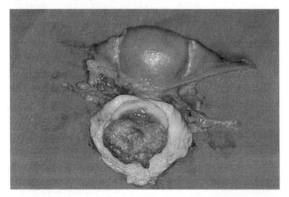

Fig. 11.3 Cervical cancer arising from the posterior lip of the cervix.

Problems associated with progressive disease in gynaecological cancers

- Primary treatment often affects **sexual function, fertility, and body image**, which may impact on coping strategies and need specialist counselling. Ovarian cancers often present late and so it may be appropriate to have specialist palliative care input from the point of diagnosis. Genetic counselling should be considered for close female relatives of patients with ovarian cancer, particularly if there is also a strong family history of breast cancer

- **Perineal and pelvic pain** is common in all three of the common gynaecological malignancies. There is nearly always a neuropathic element to the pain which may be only partially opioid sensitive

- **Lymphoedema affecting one or both limbs** develops with uncontrolled pelvic disease. It can develop at any time and frequently affects both lower limbs. It needs to be actively managed if complications are to be avoided. Management includes good skin care, avoiding additional trauma to the affected leg(s) and appropriately fitting compression garments

- **Ascites** is particularly common with ovarian cancer and can be difficult to manage. Oral diuretics, particularly spironolactone in combination with a loop diuretic such as furosemide, may help a little. Repeated paracentesis may be needed

- **Acute/sub-acute bowel obstruction** is often not amenable to surgical intervention and should be managed medically using subcutaneous medication via a syringe driver. Nasogastric tubes are rarely needed, and hydration can often be maintained orally if the nausea and vomiting are adequately controlled

- **Renal impairment** can develop in any patient with advanced pelvic disease. It may be a pre-terminal event. Ureteric stenting may be appropriate depending on the patient's perceived prognosis, the patient's wishes, and future treatment options. Renal impairment increases the risk of a patient developing opioid toxicity as renal excretion of opioid metabolites may be reduced

- **Vaginal bleeding** may respond to antifibrinolytic agents such as tranexamic acid, radiotherapy, and/or surgery

- **Offensive vaginal discharge** can cause considerable distress to both patient and carers. Topical or systemic metronidazole may help, as can barrier creams. Deodorizing machines may also help if the patient is confined to one room

- **Vesico-colic and recto-vaginal fistulae** need surgical assessment. These can be very difficult to manage and require a multidisciplinary approach

---

CASE HISTORY

PB: 'I bleed sometimes after we have intercourse'

Mrs PB is a married woman aged 32 who runs her own business. She has a 4-year-old child and, whilst she takes the combined oral contraceptive pill, plans to have another baby in the near future. For the past 4 months she has been having some light bleeding between her periods and puts this down to occasionally forgetting to take her 'pill'. On several occasions in the past 2 months she has experienced painless bleeding after sex and this has prompted her to attend her general practitioner. She is not unduly alarmed as she had a 'normal cervical smear' 3 years ago.

Her GP performs a speculum examination and sees a 2-cm warty lesion on the anterior lip of the cervix which is bleeding. She makes an immediate referral to the colposcopy clinic at the regional gynaecological cancer centre where Mrs PB is seen and a colposcopic assessment is made. This includes a cervical biopsy. When the result is available, an appointment is arranged for Mrs PB and her husband to meet the consultant gynaecological oncologist, who explains the diagnosis is cervical cancer and what investigations are required to determine the appropriate treatment.

The staging procedure involves an MRI scan of the pelvis, followed by an examination under anaesthetic, cystoscopy, and biopsy of the cervix.

The FIGO clinical stage of the tumour is 1b and at further consultation Mrs PB is offered a radical hysterectomy, which she accepts.

The operation is performed 2 weeks later without complication. The histology report indicates a completely excised squamous carcinoma with lymph channel involvement and microscopic tumour deposits in two small lymph nodes.

This finding is discussed at the multidisciplinary oncology meeting and it is decided to offer Mrs PB adjuvant radiotherapy, which she accepts. After the radiotherapy is complete, Mrs PB is reviewed at the gynaecological oncology clinic and it is apparent that she is unhappy. After a lengthy consultation, it emerges that Mrs PB has had several unanswered questions. These include: Why did my last smear not diagnose the cancer? What caused the cancer? Will it come back?

She also has fears related to running her business, sex, hormone replacement therapy, bladder and bowel functions, and expresses anger and frustration at being unable to have further children. As many of these questions as possible are answered and with the patient's permission she is referred to the oncology counselling team.

Chapter summary

Ovarian

- Ovarian cancer is the fifth commonest cancer in women (commonest gynaecological cancer in the UK)
- Risk reduced by reducing number of ovulatory cycles
- Median age at diagnosis 66 years
- Presents late with abdominal distension, abdominal pain, altered bowel habit
- 5-year survival < 40–50%
- The main treatment aim is to remove tumour surgically and follow with chemotherapy
- Patients who relapse will ultimately develop chemotherapy-resistant disease

Endometrial

- In UK affects more women than cervical cancer
- Post-menopausal disease
- Associated with obesity, low parity, late menopause, hypertension, and diabetes
- 60–70% are adenocarcinoma with degree of differentiation significant for management
- Present with post- or peri-menopausal bleeding
- Treatment: total abdominal hysterectomy and bilateral salpingo-oophorectomy (TAH and BSO) followed by radiotherapy
- Poor differentiation, myometrial invasion, lymph node metastases give an adverse prognosis

Cervix

- Second commonest female cancer worldwide
- Strong association with early intercourse, human papillomavirus (HPV) 16 (less strongly HPV 18 and 31)
- 75% are squamous in origin from cervical–columnar junction
- Screening programmes have reduced incidence, but large proportion of malignancies arise in women who have not been screened within 5 years
- Presents classically with post-coital or inter-menstrual bleeding
- Tumour invasion is by direct spread and along lymphatics
- Management in early stages is with surgery or radiotherapy
- Chemo-radiotherapy is used in women with more advanced disease

Palliative issues

- Particularly challenging because of issues relating to sexuality, body image, and fertility
- Perineal and pelvic pain is complex and difficult to manage
- Ascites, bowel obstruction, renal impairment, offensive discharge, lymphoedema, vesico-vaginal and vesico-colic fistulae require a multiprofessional approach

References

1. http://info.cancerresearchuk.org/cancerstats/types/ovary/incidence/
2. http://info.cancerresearchuk.org/cancerstats/types/ovary/mortality/
3. http://info.cancerresearchuk.org/cancerstats/types/uterus/incidence/
4. http://info.cancerresearchuk.org/cancerstats/types/uterus/mortality/
5. http://info.cancerresearchuk.org/cancerstats/types/cervix/incidence/
6. http://info.cancerresearchuk.org/cancerstats/types/cervix/mortality/

CHAPTER 12

Patients with upper gastrointestinal cancers

Oesophageal carcinoma

Incidence and mortality

In 2001 4,682 men and 2,793 women were diagnosed with oesophageal cancer in the UK.[1]

In 2003 4,740 men and 2,610 women died from oesophageal cancer in the UK.[2]

Background

- Eighth most commonly occurring cancer in the UK (7,000 new patients each year in the UK)
- More common in men than women (2 : 1)
- Tumours in the upper two-thirds of the oesophagus are usually squamous cell cancers; incidence of these squamous cell tumours is stable
- Tumours in the lower one-third are predominantly adenocarcinoma; incidence of adenocarcinoma has been steadily increasing
- Adenocarcinoma often arises in a Barrett's oesophagus (glandular metaplasia of squamous cell lining of lower third of oesophagus usually related to gastro-oesophageal reflux); endoscopic screening may reduce the incidence
- Second most common site for small cell carcinoma – up to 2% of all oesophageal cancers
- Overall survival in the UK is < 10% at 5 years

Oesophageal tumour characteristics

- Expand circumferentially and also extend submucosally
- Involvement of mediastinal structures (trachea, pleura, pericardium, major vessels) occurs but not commonly

---

Key Facts

Risk factors for oesophageal carcinoma

- Excessive alcohol consumption
- Smoking
- Barrett's oesophagus
- Vitamin-deficient diet
- Patterson–Brown–Kelly syndrome
- Tylosis

- Common sites of lymphatic spread dependent on primary site of tumour:
  - Upper one-third of oesophagus to supraclavicular and cervical nodes
  - Middle third to mediastinum
  - Lower third to coeliac nodes
- More distant nodal spread considered metastatic disease

Key Facts

- Upper one-third < 10% (mostly squamous carcinoma)
- Middle one-third 40% (mostly squamous carcinoma)
- Lower one-third 50% (> 50% adenocarcinoma, remainder squamous)

Symptoms

- Dysphagia
- Chest pain
- Dyspepsia
- Weight loss

Investigations

Endoscopy is the diagnostic investigation of choice for all middle-aged or elderly patients with dysphagia as it allows biopsy of suspicious lesions.

Diagnosis and staging

- Endoscopy and biopsy
- Barium swallow – demonstrates tumour length
- Endoluminal ultrasound – demonstrates extent of local invasion and lymph node involvement
- Computerized tomography (CT) scan – assesses nodal involvement and distant metastases
- Laparoscopy should be performed in potentially operable tumours
- Bronchoscopy should be performed if tracheal involvement is suspected
- Positron emission tomography scanning is used increasingly in staging to detect involved nodes and distant metastases. Because of PET, fewer oesophagal resections are being performed.

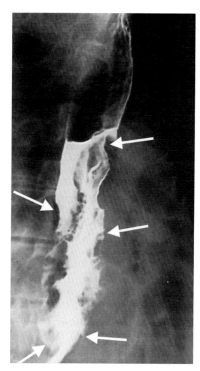

Fig. 12.1 Barium swallow demonstrating extensive adenocarcinoma in the lower third of the oesophagus.

Key Fact

One in three patients presenting with oesophageal cancer is suitable for surgery. http://www.cancer-help.org.uk/

Treatment

Resectable disease

Patients who are suitable for radical surgery do substantially better than those who are not. This is complex surgery best done by a specialized team. Surgery remains the only potentially curative modality for tumours in the lower two-thirds of oesophagus. By contrast, surgery is usually not appropriate for patients with tumours of the upper third, which require management in collaboration with specialist head and neck surgeons and oncologists.

Unfortunately as a result of the tendency of oesophageal tumours to spread longitudinally through the submucosa, circumferentially to other mediastinal structures, and to lymph nodes early in their course, the results from surgery are disappointing.

◆ Node negative resection 5-year survival 40–57%

◆ Node positive resection 5-year survival 8–23%

◆ Overall survival rate in patients with surgery at 5 years 20%

◆ Overall survival without surgery at 5 years < 10%

◆ Neo-adjuvant chemotherapy with cisplatin and 5-fluorouracil improves resectability and reduces the likelihood of local and distant relapse. Studies have not as yet established that the increased morbidity is justified in terms of response and survival benefits

◆ Chemoradiotherapy may also be used with radical intent in tumours in the lower two-thirds of oesophagus in patients with localized disease who are unfit for surgery

Unresectable disease

Endoscopic placement of stents or radiotherapy may provide palliation.

Platinum-based chemotherapy may also be useful in palliating symptoms of dysphagia in patients who are

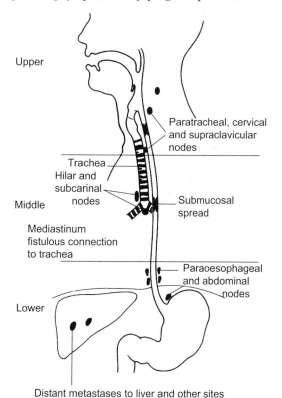

Fig. 12.2 Local and distant spread of oesophageal cancer. Reproduced with permission from Souhami and Tobias, *Cancer and its management*, 3e, Blackwell Publishing.

fit. Squamous carcinomas have response rates in the order of 50% to cisplatin and 5-fluorouracil combinations. Adenocarcinoma of the gastro-oesophageal junction has a > 50% response rate to ECF (epirubicin, cisplatin, 5-fluorouracil).

CASE HISTORY

JR: 'I just can't swallow'

A 70-year-old woman, JR, reported increasing dysphagia which she localized to an area about 3 cm below her manubrium sternae. She had lost 8 kg in weight over 9 months. Dysphagia was progressive and when seen at outpatients she could swallow only fluids.

Barium swallow showed a stricture extending from 5 cm below the level of the carina to just above the diaphragm. Endoscopy revealed a malignant stricture and biopsy was positive for adenocarcinoma. Staging CT scan showed no evidence of metastatic disease and she underwent a total thoracic oesophagectomy with her stomach drawn up through the mediastinum and anastomosed.

She experienced considerable difficulties obtaining adequate nutrition after surgery, but had dietetic advice and consumed high-calorie food supplements. She eventually gained weight to just 2 kg less than her previous weight and is well 3 years later, having had a benign stricture at her anastomosis dilated 8 months after her surgery.

Comment

This woman's characteristic symptoms of weight loss with significant dysphagia, which resulted in weight loss as a result of calorie restriction, are typical of oesophageal carcinoma. The differential diagnosis includes benign oesophageal strictures, and endoscopy and biopsy are required to establish the diagnosis. Assessment of the tumour for operability is very important as surgery is the only clearly recognized therapy resulting in long-term survival or cure. However, the majority of patients treated surgically will still relapse despite initially successful treatment. In this case the patient required nutritional advice and support to regain weight, even after surgery.

Stomach cancer

Incidence and mortality

In 2001 5,790 men and 3,314 women were diagnosed with stomach cancer in the UK.[3]

In 2003 3,744 men and 2,273 women died from stomach cancer in the UK.[4]

Background

- Sixth most common cancer in the UK

- Very high incidence in Japan and Korea (where endoscopic surveillance programmes have been introduced), Central and South America, and Eastern Europe

- In the UK incidence of cancer of the distal stomach is falling but the incidence of tumours of the cardia or gastro-oesophageal junction is rising

- More common in men than women (2 : 1), in lower socioeconomic groups, and in those over 60 years of age

- Associated with:
  - *Helicobacter pylori* infection
  - Atrophic gastritis
  - Achlorhydria
  - Pernicious anaemia
  - Blood group A

- 90–95% of gastric tumours are adenocarcinoma

- Half of stomach tumours arise in the pyloric region, most of the rest on the lesser curve

- Tumours spread longitudinally, submucosally, and circumferentially, invading muscle layers and adjacent structures or lymphatically to coeliac nodes

- Transcoelomic spread leads to peritoneal seedlings and tumour deposits in ovaries (Krukenberg tumours) may occur

- Haematogenous spread via the portal system to liver or systemic circulation to lung, brain, bone, and skin

- Gastric lymphoma may present in a similar manner but is a very different disease, requiring different management and with a different prognosis

- Other rarer cancers arising in the stomach include neuroendocrine cancers and gastrointestinal stromal tumours (GIST) which are also treated differently from adenocarcinomas

Prognosis

> **Key Fact**
>
> Because most stomach cancer is advanced when detected the overall 5-year survival is only 20%.
> http://www.cancerhelp.org.uk

In patients who have had radical surgery:

- Disease confined to mucosa alone (very uncommon) – 5-year survival approaches 100%
- Node negative patients without serosal involvement – 5-year survival 50%
- Lymph node involvement or involvement of serosa – 5-year survival 17–31%

Signs and symptoms

- Insidious onset
- Anaemia
- Early satiety and anorexia
- Weight loss
- Dyspepsia

Clinical examination may reveal an epigastric mass or lymphatic spread may present with an enlarged left supraclavicular fossa node (Troisier's sign).

Investigation

Endoscopy is the diagnostic investigation of choice allowing direct visualization and biopsy.

Diagnosis and staging

- *Full staging is essential if inappropriate surgery is to be avoided*
- Endoscopy and biopsy
- Endoluminal ultrasound to assess depth of invasion and lymph node involvement

> **Test Yourself**
>
> **Helicobacter and cancer control**
> How would you devise a study to show if a world-wide approach to preventing *Helicobacter* infection would have significant impact on the incidence of upper gastrointestinal malignancy?

- CT scan to assess lymph node involvement and distant metastases
- Laparoscopy – may be indicated to assess peritoneal or liver disease if surgery is being considered; laparoscopic ultrasound is particularly useful to detect and biopsy possible liver metastases

Treatment

Resectable disease

Surgery remains the only potentially curative modality of treatment. Partial or total gastrectomy (depending on tumour site and mode of spread) with regional lymphadenectomy is the most commonly performed operation. Factors determining outcome include:

- Tumour location – patients with distal tumours do better than those with more proximally located tumours
- Tumour extent – patients with tumours beyond the gastric wall have a worse prognosis
- Extent of lymph node involvement: the Japanese have excellent results with extensive lymph node dissection but these have not been replicated in the West

Following surgery many patients remain at high risk of local and distant disease relapse. Trials have suggested that such patients may benefit from adjuvant chemotherapy or chemoradiation.

Combined pre and post-operative chemotherapy has been shown to increase resectability and reduce relapse rates in patients with operable gastric cancer.

Locally advanced/metastatic disease

Palliative operations can be performed to control pain or bleeding or to relieve obstruction for patients with advanced disease. The type of operation performed depends to a large extent on the performance status of the patient and the anticipated disease course.

Chemotherapy, with combinations of cisplatin and 5-fluorouracil with or without epirubicin, also has palliative benefit for patients with locally advanced or metastatic gastric cancer and may also improve survival by some months. Trials to determine the role of oxaliplatin, irinotecan, taxanes, and oral fluoropyrimidines in the palliative treatment of advanced gastric cancer are showing encouraging results.

Endoscopic procedures such as stenting or laser coagulation may also provide useful palliative benefits.

Very occasionally radiotherapy may provide useful palliation, e.g. for bleeding from locally advanced

Test Yourself

JD: 'The weight is just dropping off me'

Mr JD is a 69-year-old man who reported anorexia and weight loss of 12 kg over the past 3 months. He has had epigastric pain and a feeling of early satiety over the past month. He also reported that he has had poor energy over the last 6 months. He had vomited twice in the last 24 hours with the vomitus on both occasions containing dark brown material. He has also had three angina attacks in the past 2 days.

Medical history

Myocardial infarction 5 years ago and poorly controlled angina since. He has had two hospital admissions for bronchopneumonia in the past year.

Family and social history

He lives alone and has no immediate family alive. He smokes 20 cigarettes per day and is a retired farm labourer.

Medications

He takes nifedipine 20 mg four times daily and glyceryl trinitrate spray prn. He has recently finished a course of antibiotics for 'bronchitis'.

On examination

Pale. Blood pressure 98/56 mmHg, pulse 98 bpm. Palpable 2-cm left supraclavicular lymph node. Chest clear.

Abdominal examination reveals an ill-defined epigastric mass which is slightly tender. He has an enlarged liver palpated at five finger breadths in the mid-clavicular line. No other positive findings recorded.

After initial treatment, a fibre-optic upper gastrointestinal endoscopy shows a 10 × 8-cm tumour mass on the lesser curvature of the stomach near the pylorus and a large amount of food residue in the stomach despite adequate preparation. Biopsy reveals an adenocarcinoma. Fine needle aspiration of the supraclavicular fossa node also demonstrates malignant cells similar to those seen on the stomach biopsy.

Questions

1. What are the presenting symptoms for stomach cancer?
2. What was the 'initial treatment'?
3. Why did this man develop vomiting?
4. What are the therapeutic options for him?

tumours. It may also be useful in palliating pain caused by metastatic disease, e.g. bone metastases.

The rare GISTs have aroused much therapeutic interest with the dramatic impact ('The huge lump in my tummy just disappeared') of biological therapy with imatinib (Glivec®) in *some* patients, see page 47.

Pancreatic carcinoma

Incidence and mortality

In 2001 3,332 men and 3,586 women were diagnosed with pancreatic cancer in the UK.[5]

In 2003 3,421 men and 2,619 women died from pancreatic cancer in the UK.[6]

Background

♦ Seventh most common cause of cancer death in the UK
♦ Predominantly 60–80 years age group
♦ 75% arise from the head of the pancreas, 15% from the body, and 10% from the tail
♦ Risk factors include:
  • Smoking
  • Chronic pancreatitis
  • Animal fats in diet
  • Previous surgery for peptic ulcer disease
  • Alcohol
♦ Protective factors:
  • Citrus fruits
  • Vegetables
♦ 90% are adenocarcinoma

Presentation

Symptom onset may be insidious – especially for tumours in body and tail of the pancreas.

♦ Jaundice
♦ Anorexia
♦ Weight loss
♦ Pain – local invasion of tail or body tumours may cause severe abdominal pain radiating to the back
♦ Paraneoplastic features e.g. migratory thrombophlebitis; hypercoagulable syndrome (deep vein thrombosis; pulmonary thromboembolism)

- Pancreatic head tumours may present with painless jaundice as a consequence of common bile duct obstruction

- Malabsorption and steatorrhoea may arise from biliary obstruction or pancreatic insufficiency caused by tumour infiltration or atrophy of normal pancreas

- 10% of patients will develop diabetes mellitus

Investigations

- Biochemical:
  - Liver function tests may show an obstructive pattern
  - CA 19-9 is elevated in the majority of cancers but is not sufficiently sensitive or specific to be diagnostic alone

- Endoscopic:
  - Endoscopic retrograde cholangiopancreatography (ERCP) allows assessment and stenting of obstructed bile duct
  - Endoluminal ultrasound allows assessment of the pancreatic head and its relationship to surrounding blood vessels as well as tissue biopsy

- Radiological:
  - Ultrasound scan or CT with fine-needle aspiration or biopsy of pancreatic mass
  - CT chest abdomen and pelvis
  - Magnetic resonance imaging (MRI) can delineate tumour, ducts and vessels with less morbidity than ERCP

- Laparoscopy:
  - May be required to assess peritoneal involvement prior to surgery

Management

Surgery is the only potentially curative modality of treatment.

Unfortunately, less than 15% of patients present with surgically resectable disease.

A pancreaticoduodenectomy (originally described by Whipple) is the operation of choice. Such complex surgery should only be carried out by specialized surgical teams to optimize results.

Even in those patients who are suitable candidates for this surgery 5-year survival is less than 10%.

The majority of patients will present with advanced unresectable disease, although surgical bypass procedures may be possible.

If presenting with biliary obstruction, primary treatment is aimed at relief of jaundice, which is generally achieved by endoscopic or percutaneous transhepatic stent placement.

Patients with persistent back pain may benefit from intra-operative or percutaneous coeliac axis block by alcohol injection, or local radiotherapy to the area of retroperitoneal tumour invasion.

Pancreatic enzyme supplements may help with malabsorption.

Chemotherapy with gemcitabine can provide a modest survival benefit and should be considered in patients with unresectable disease and an Eastern Cooperative Oncology Group performance status of less than 3.

Addition of the oral fluoropyrimidine capecitabine to gemcitabine may further prolong survival.

Addition of the anti-epidermal growth factor receptor tyrosine kinase inhibitor erlotinib to gemcitabine may also improve survival over gemcitabine alone, but by only a small amount.

Hepatoma (hepatocellular cancer)

Incidence and mortality

Hepatoma (hepatocellular cancer) is rare in the UK where there are approximately 100 new cases per year and approximately the same number of deaths. There is a slight male predominance.

> **Key Fact**
>
> Hepatoma is the most common tumour worldwide with approximately one million cases occurring each year.

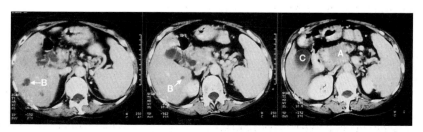

Fig. 12.3 Cancer of the head of pancreas. CT scan demonstrating (A) mass in head of pancreas, (B) dilated intrahepatic bile ducts, and (C) dilated gallbladder (clinically palpable as Courvoisier's sign).

There is geographical variation, with high incidence in certain areas of Asia and Africa where hepatitis B is endemic.

Aetiology

The most clearly defined predisposing factor for hepatoma is cirrhosis of the liver, which is present in 80% of cases. Cirrhosis can be the result of hepatitis B or C, alcohol, haemochromatosis, chronic active hepatitis, and other less common causes.

Hepatic toxins can also cause hepatoma. Aflatoxin, the mycotoxin produced by *Aspergillus flavus*, is found in stored cereals in tropical climates and is a significant hepatic carcinogen.

Pathology

Hepatomas often arise from regenerating nodules in a cirrhotic liver and may be multifocal.

The tumour cells characteristically secrete oncofetal protein (α-fetoprotein), which can serve as a tumour marker for the disease but is not specific for hepatoma.

Tumour cells invade the portal venous system or ducts and therefore intrahepatic spread is common and early in this disease. Tumour will also invade through the liver capsule into adjacent structures. Lymph nodes adjacent to the liver are commonly involved, and it may also spread via lymphatics and via the bloodstream. Lung and bone are common systemic sites of spread.

Presentation

Patients with hepatoma often have a known diagnosis of cirrhosis and associated liver problems. The development of the hepatoma may lead to increasing anorexia and weight loss. Pain in the epigastrium may occur as a result of distension of the liver capsule. Haemorrhage into the capsule may cause acute pain, with peritonitis or pleurisy. Most patients will have hepatomegaly with either diffuse enlargement or the presence of a sizeable mass. An arterial bruit and hepatic rub may be heard over the tumour. Compression of the inferior vena cava and liver impairment may lead to leg oedema and ascites. The liver may be diffusely enlarged, or there may be a palpable mass caused by the hepatoma or by cirrhosis. In the differential diagnosis of a focal mass or multiple masses in the liver, one must exclude metastatic deposits from a primary cancer elsewhere.

A sizeable hepatoma can secrete an insulin-like peptide and give rise to hypoglycaemia.

Tumour may also secrete parathormone, giving rise to hypercalcaemia, or oestrogens, giving rise to feminization. If portal vein thrombosis occurs, then splenomegaly and oesophageal varices may develop.

Investigations

Ultrasound, angiography, CT scanning, and magnetic resonance imaging all contribute useful information regarding operability of the tumour. They will also facilitate a fine-needle biopsy where the status of coagulation factors permits.

Treatment

Less than 15% of patients will be suitable for radical surgery.

If the tumour proves inoperable, then benefit can be obtained from ligation of the hepatic artery, which supplies a vast majority of the circulation to the hepatoma. If the portal vein is obstructed then ischaemic necrosis of the liver is also possible.

Unfortunately, collateral circulation will develop after hepatic artery embolization and this is essentially short-term palliation for a sizeable tumour mass.

Hepatic artery embolization is an alternative procedure. This can be more selective, causing fewer untoward symptoms. Chemotherapeutic agents can also be infused through the hepatic artery, with increased retention in the liver if embolization is performed at the same time. Embolization can also be repeated at future dates. If significant systemic symptoms arise from metastatic disease, anthracycline-based chemotherapy (doxorubicin) may be considered as a palliative measure.

Prognosis

Overall, for hepatoma patients, median survival is less than 3 months for patients with cirrhosis and approaching 1 year in patients without cirrhosis. In the UK, only 5% of patients with cirrhosis and 50% of patients without cirrhosis have resectable tumours.

Key Fact

Metastases in the setting of liver cirrhosis are extremely rare and raised serum α-fetoprotein supports the diagnosis of hepatoma.

Stop and Think

The most important aetiological factor worldwide is hepatitis B infection and widespread vaccination against hepatitis B virus would dramatically reduce the incidence of hepatoma.

Why is this not happening?

Problems associated with progressive disease in patients with upper gastrointestinal cancer

Mild and non-specific symptoms often precede the onset of dysphagia for many months in oesophageal carcinoma. Stomach cancer often presents late and is frequently metastatic at presentation.

- **Liver capsule pain** as a result of liver metastases is common. This is only partially opioid-responsive but responds well to non-steroidal anti-inflammatory drugs or oral steroids

- **Oesophageal spasm** may occur and can be difficult to manage. It may be aggravated by oesophageal candidiasis, which needs systemic treatment with oral antifungal drugs. Smooth muscle relaxants such as nifedipine may also help. The palliative care team can often help with managing such symptoms

- **Involvement of the coeliac plexus** causes a difficult pain syndrome with non-specific abdominal pain and mid-back pain. Blockade of the plexus using anaesthetic techniques can be useful

- **Dysphagia** can occur in both oesophageal and stomach cancer. It may be helped by stenting. Oncological treatment of the tumour may provide temporary relief. Advice about appropriate diet and consistency of the food may also help. A feeding gastrostomy is occasionally used before aggressive treatment to improve functional status and the ability to tolerate such an intervention. A gastrostomy can also improve nutrition and quality of life but should only be inserted after careful multidisciplinary discussion involving the patient and family. Ethical dilemmas can arise towards the end of life when issues of avoiding the prolongation of an uncomfortable dying period (by reducing or stopping artificial feeding) may need to be discussed. There is no evidence that the insertion of feeding tubes in the dying either extends life or improves symptoms

- **Anorexia** is frequent and often profound. There may be a fear of eating because of pain. This may bring the patient and their carer into conflict about food and the 'need to eat'. Open and honest explanation can help to relieve anxiety and provide practical approaches to dealing with the situation

- **Weight loss and altered body image** can be profound with these cancers and can cause distressing problems for the patient and their family

- **Nausea and vomiting** can be persistent and difficult to control. Specialist advice is often needed and drugs may need to be given by routes other than oral. Small frequent meals may reduce the frequency of vomiting

- **Haematemesis** may be one of the presenting symptoms but can also occur as the tumour progresses. Where possible local treatment may help and brachytherapy and laser therapy, where available, can reduce the incidence. There is risk of a major bleed. This is a difficult situation to manage and early involvement of the palliative care team should be considered

Chapter summary
Oesophageal carcinoma

- Eighth most commonly occurring cancer in the UK
- Tumours in the upper two-thirds of oesophagus are usually squamous cell cancers
- Tumours in the lower third are predominantly adenocarcinoma
- Overall survival in the UK is < 10% at 5 years
- Endoluminal ultrasound demonstrates extent of local invasion and lymph node involvement
- Endoscopic placement of stents or radiotherapy may provide palliation, as may chemotherapy

Stomach carcinoma

- Sixth most common cancer in the UK
- Associated with:
  - *Helicobacter pylori* infection
  - Atrophic gastritis
  - Achlorhydria
  - Pernicious anaemia
  - Blood group A
- Full staging is essential if inappropriate surgery is to be avoided
- Partial or total gastrectomy (depending on tumour site and mode of spread) and regional lymphadenectomy is the most commonly performed surgery
- Palliative operations can be performed to control pain or bleeding or to relieve obstruction for patients with advanced disease
- Chemotherapy may relieve symptoms and prolong survival

Chapter summary—*cont'd.*

- Chemotherapy may also have palliative benefit for patients with locally advanced or metastatic gastric carcinoma.

- Radiotherapy may provide useful palliation

Pancreatic carcinoma

- Seventh most common cause of cancer death in the UK

- 75% arise from the head of pancreas, 15% from the body, 10% from the tail

- Risk factors include: smoking, alcohol, chronic pancreatitis, diabetes mellitus, animal fats in diet, previous surgery for peptic ulcer disease

- Presentation: *Insidious onset of symptoms,* jaundice, weight loss, backache

- Less than 15% of patients present with surgically resectable disease

- Chemotherapy including gemcitabine provides a small survival benefit in selected patients

Hepatoma

- Hepatoma (hepatocellular cancer) is rare in the UK

- Hepatoma is the most common tumour world-wide with approximately one million cases occuring each year

- The most clearly defined predisposing factor for hepatoma is cirrhosis of the liver

- Cirrhosis can be due to hepatitis B or C, alcohol, haemochromatosis, chronic active hepatitis, and other less common causes

- Metastases in the setting of liver cirrhosis are extremely rare and raised serum α-fetoprotein supports the diagnosis of hepatoma

- Overall, median survival is less than 3 months for patients with cirrhosis and approaching 1 year in patients without cirrhosis

References

1. http://info.cancerresearchuk.org/cancerstats/types/oesophagus/incidence/
2. http://info.cancerresearchuk.org/cancerstats/types/oesophagus/mortality/
3. http://info.cancerresearchuk.org/cancerstats/types/stomach/incidence/
4. http://info.cancerresearchuk.org/cancerstats/types/stomach/mortality/
5. http://info.cancerresearchuk.org/cancerstats/types/pancreas/incidence/
6. http://info.cancerresearchuk.org/cancerstats/types/pancreas/mortality/

Patients with genitourinary cancers

Incidence

In the UK in 2001 the following genitourinary malignancies were diagnosed.

TABLE 13.1 Incidence of genitourinary cancers by gender

	Men	Women
Prostate	30,142	–
Kidney	3,842	2,318
Bladder	7,581	3,078
Testicular	1,996	–

- The incidence of all types of genitourinary malignancy is increasing

- This is partly the result of increased numbers of elderly people in the population and improvements in diagnostic techniques, but there has been a significant increase in the incidence of renal, prostatic, and testicular cancer

- Environmental exposure to carcinogens may account for the increase in testicular cancer

- The outlook for patients with genitourinary malignancy is improving

Prostate cancer

Incidence and mortality

In 2001 30,142 men were diagnosed with prostate cancer in the UK.[1]

In 2003 10,164 men died from prostate cancer in the UK.[2]

Background

- Accounts for approximately 30% of all cancers in men

- Second only to lung cancer as a cause of cancer deaths in men

Risk factors

- Increasing age is major risk factor – 70% of men > 80 years old have some evidence of prostatic cancer at post mortem
- Appears to be linked to androgen exposure – rare in men castrated before 40 years of age
- Race – high incidence in northern Europe, North America; low in Far Eastern countries; more common in black population than white
- Genetic – two- to threefold increase if first-degree relative is affected
- Incidence of prostate cancer is rising – in part this is the result of increased detection of early disease by prostate-specific antigen (PSA) screening
- The lifetime risk of developing prostate cancer is 30%, but only 10% of cancers will be clinically significant

Presentation

- Urinary outflow symptoms, e.g. frequency, nocturia (indistinguishable from benign prostatic enlargement)
- Symptoms of metastatic disease, bone pain, sciatica, anaemia, weight loss and, less commonly, lymphoedema
- Raised PSA can be a marker of prostate cancer. There are, however, other causes of a raised PSA. Moreover, many patients with a raised PSA and prostate cancer will not become symptomatic

Grading of prostate cancer

The Gleason system is based on the degree of glandular differentiation (Gleason grade 1 is well differentiated, and grade 5 is poorly differentiated) which is closely associated with disease progression.

Diagnosis and staging

Patients with raised PSA or palpable prostate abnormalities are evaluated by transurethral ultrasound (TRUS), and local biopsy.

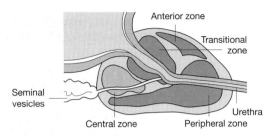

Key Facts

Prostate cancer survival rates

One-year survival rates		Five-year survival rates	
1971–75	1996–99	1971–75	1996–99
65%	87%	31%	65%

Anterior zone
Transitional zone
Seminal vesicles
Urethra
Central zone
Peripheral zone
70% of cancers arise in the peripheral zone
15–20% arise in the transitional zone
15–20% arise in the central zone
Cancers are often multifocal, > 97% are adenocarcinomas from prostatic acinar cells

Fig. 13.1 Anatomy.

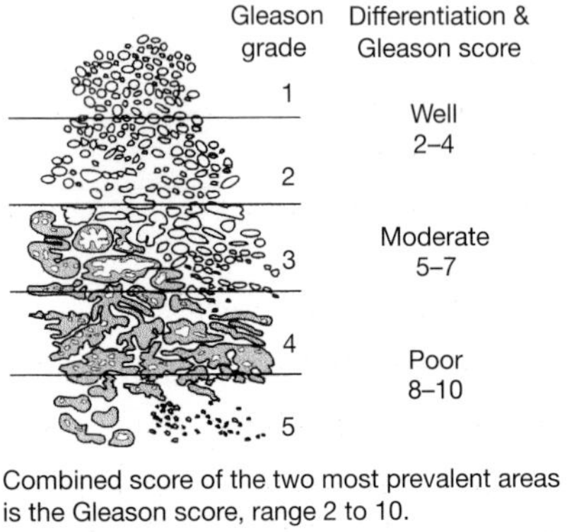

Gleason grade
Differentiation & Gleason score
1
2
3
4
5
Well 2–4
Moderate 5–7
Poor 8–10
Combined score of the two most prevalent areas is the Gleason score, range 2 to 10.

Fig. 13.2 Pathology.

TABLE 13.2 Gleason scores and outcome

Gleason score	Differentiation	% Likelihood of local progression by 10 years	% Likelihood of death from cancer by 15 years
2–4	Well	25	8
5–7	Moderate	50	35
8–10	Poor	70	65

Key Facts

Causes of an elevated PSA

- Benign prostatic hyperplasia
- Prostate cancer
- Prostate infection
- Prostate biopsy

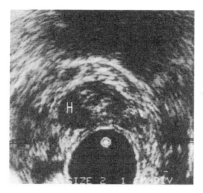

Fig. 13.3 TRUS image of prostate. Biopsy of hypoechoic region H is performed using the TRUS probe with biopsy needle mounted.

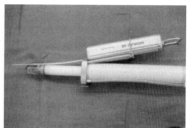

- **Digital rectal examination** provides information on the size of the prostate and changes in texture and architecture but is examiner dependent

- Many older men have a raised PSA but are asymptomatic and will not die of their disease, even if there is an underlying cancer

- **PSA assessment:** PSA is a glycoprotein secreted by prostatic cells

  - PSA > 4 ng/ml: clinical suspicion
  - PSA 11–20 ng/ml: 66% of patients have cancer
  - PSA> 50 ng/ml: often distant bone metastases

- **Transurethral ultrasound and biopsy** are routine investigations for patients with raised PSA and/or clinical evidence of prostate cancer

- **Computerized tomography (CT) and/or magnetic resonance imaging (MRI)** may help to assess lymph node involvement

- **Isotope bone scan** if bone metastases are suspected

Management

Many prostate tumours are clinically insignificant and will not cause symptoms in the patient's lifetime. It is important, however, to recognize those patients whose tumours are likely to become clinically apparent.

Prognostic factors in patients with cancer confined to the prostate:

- Tumour grade – assessed by Gleason score
- Tumour stage – assessed clinically and radiologically
- Patient age – younger patients are more likely to develop problems than older patients

Cancer confined to the prostate gland

If aged < 70 years and fit

Consider radical local therapy, e.g.

- Prostatectomy (increasingly by laparoscopic route)
- Radiotherapy (external beam or brachytherapy)

There are currently no trial results directly comparing these approaches. In general terms, fitter patients tend to be treated with surgery rather than radiotherapy, despite the higher incidence of complications and absence of evidence of improved survival.

> **Key Facts**
>
> Brachytherapy involves the placement of radioactive sources ('seeds' or wires) either in tumours (interstitial implants) or near tumours (intracavitary therapy and mould therapy). High-dose radiation is emitted for a short distance around the source, unlike external beam radiotherapy, where radiation must traverse normal tissue to reach the tumour. The word 'brachytherapy' means 'short therapy'.

Complications:

- Prostatectomy: 50% impotence; 8–15% long-term incontinence
- Radiotherapy: 25–35% impotence; rectal bleeding/bladder irritation and bleeding (5%) but usually no incontinence (1%)

> **Key Facts**
>
> TNM staging of prostate cancer
> T_1 – Clinically inapparent
> T_2 – Palpable tumour confined to prostate
> T_3 – Tumour extends through capsule
> T_4 – Tumour is fixed or invades structures other than seminal vesicles
> N_0 – No regional nodes
> N_1 – Regional lymph node metastases
> M_0 – No metastases
> M_1 – Metastases present

If over 70 years or unfit

♦ 'Wait and see' policy

♦ Active process of examining patient regularly and treating if any suggestion of disease progression

Locally extensive disease (T₃/T₄)

Locally extensive disease (T_3/T_4)

♦ Neo-adjuvant anti-androgen therapy

♦ Radical radiotherapy

Nodal disease

♦ Hormones are the mainstay of treatment

Distant metastatic disease

♦ The natural history is very variable with a number of patients with metastatic bone disease living for > 5 years following diagnosis (median survival 4 years)

♦ The majority of tumours are sensitive to androgens. Hormonal manipulation aimed at reducing the effect of androgens (mainly testosterone) at a cellular level will produce responses in around 70% of men with bone metastases with a median response duration of 12–18 months

♦ Commonly used hormonal treatments include:

  • Medical castration with luteinizing hormone releasing hormone (LHRH) agonists. (These can induce a flare of hormone-induced activity on initiating therapy, which needs to be suppressed with anti-androgens for 1 week prior to treatment and the initial 2 weeks of treatment)

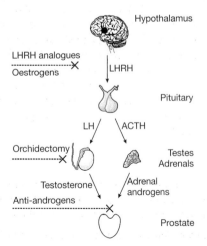

Fig. 13.4 Pituitary, testicular and adrenal axis showing the major sites of hormone blockade (LHRH, luteinizing hormone releasing hormone; LH, luteinizing hormone; ACTH, adrenocorticotrophic hormone).

• Anti-androgens (cyproterone acetate, flutamide, bicalutamide): these may be used alone or in combination with LHRH analogues. The value of the combination, however, is uncertain

• The oestrogen stilboestrol may be used after other hormones have failed. This is given in a lower dose than in the past, to minimize thromboembolic side effects

• Bilateral orchidectomy is less popular because of the availability of medical methods of castration

The side effects of these hormone treatments include:

♦ Loss of libido and potency

♦ Hot flushes

♦ Change in fat deposition

♦ Osteoporosis

♦ Poor concentration

♦ Decreased energy and drive

Local radiotherapy may be useful as an additional palliative measure particularly for bone pain; Strontium[89], a bone-seeking radioisotope (intravenous), is an effective but expensive treatment for reducing bone pain.

Hormone refractory prostate cancer

The prognosis for patients whose disease has progressed through anti-androgen therapy is poor.

Therapeutic options at this stage include:

♦ Anti-androgen withdrawal – this results in a response in a small number of patients

♦ Chemotherapy – prostate cancer is relatively chemoresistant and no standard regimen has been established. Mitoxantrone and prednisolone, however, have been used to palliate symptoms. Docetaxel has produced an increase in median survival of 2 months but is appropriate only for fitter patients

Problems associated with progressive disease in prostate cancer

♦ **Pathological fracture.** This may occur without obvious trauma. It may need orthopaedic intervention (pinning or joint replacement) and radiotherapy. Prophylactic orthopaedic intervention may also be required for bone lesions at high risk of fracture

♦ **Spinal cord compression** requires prompt diagnosis and treatment with high-dose steroids and usually radiotherapy. A minority of cases may be suitable for surgical intervention; such patients include those with a single site of disease

♦ **Neuropathic pain**. Local recurrence of tumour, pelvic spread or a collapsed vertebra may cause neuropathic pain. Such pain is partially opioid sensitive but adjuvant analgesics are usually required to supplement the effect of the opioid

♦ **Bone pain**. Specialist advice should be sought about the appropriate use of radiotherapy and radioactive strontium as well as nerve blockade. Bisphosphonates such as pamidronate and zoledronate help to reduce bone pain and also reduce the number of cancer-associated skeletal events and the incidence of hypercalcaemia

♦ **Bone marrow failure** may occur in patients with advanced disease. Typically the patient has symptomatic anaemia and thrombocytopenia. Palliative blood transfusions may be appropriate initially but their appropriateness should be discussed with the patient and his family when they no longer give symptomatic benefit

♦ **Retention of urine**. Problems with micturition, including haematuria, may lead to retention of urine. This may be acute and painful, or chronic and painless. If the patient is unfit for transurethral resection of the prostate, then a permanent indwelling urinary catheter should be considered. Chronic urinary retention can lead to renal failure

♦ **Lymphoedema** of the lower limbs and occasionally the genital area is usually the result of advanced pelvic disease. It needs to be actively managed by lymphoedema experts if its miserable effects are to be minimized

Altered body image and sexual dysfunction can result from hormone manipulation, radiotherapy, or surgery. This may be exacerbated by apathy and clinical depression. Specialist mental and psychological health strategies may be required.

 Case studies and multiple choice questions at www.oxfordtextbooks.co.uk/orc/watson/

Renal carcinoma

Incidence and mortality

In 2001 3,842 men and 2,318 women were diagnosed with renal cancer in the UK.[3]

In 2003 2,076 men and 1,337 women died from renal cancer in the UK.[4]

Background

♦ Renal carcinoma accounts for only 3% of all adult malignancies

---

CASE HISTORY

PB: Cancer of the prostate

A 69-year-old man, PB, presented with lower urinary tract symptoms and pain in his low back. He also complained of increasing lethargy for 3 months.

Physical examination was unremarkable but on digital rectal examination there was a hard suspicious nodule involving the right lobe of the prostate with obliteration of the median and lateral sulcus of the gland.

Investigation

Urinalysis revealed a trace of blood. His haemoglobin was 10 g/dl and creatinine was 190 mmol/l.

Serum PSA was 380 pg/ml. X-ray of dorsal and lumbar spine revealed sclerotic changes in the D_{10}–L_1 vertebrae. Ultrasound examination of the kidneys showed mild bilateral hydronephrosis. A needle biopsy of the prostate was performed under antibiotic cover.

Histology confirmed the presence of a Gleason score 7 carcinoma.

Staging

An isotope bone scan revealed multiple areas of increased uptake in the axial skeleton and ribs.

Treatment

The patient was commenced on cyproterone acetate 100 mg t.i.d. for 3 weeks and 5 days later was given an LHRH analogue subcutaneously. The patient was told that it would take several weeks for the treatment to take effect and that he might experience facial flushing and sweating as well as weight gain in the upper body. At review 3 months later his PSA level was 14, his pain and urinary tract symptoms had settled as had his hydronephrosis. He was told of the tumour response, advised to continue treatment, and given a further appointment for 4 months.

♦ The majority (85%) of malignant tumours of the kidney are renal cell carcinomas (RCC), which are thought to arise from proximal renal tubular cells

♦ Secondary deposits from lung and breast may involve the kidney on rare occasions

♦ RCC is more common in men (male : female ratio 2 : 1), occurring in the fifth and sixth decades

- The incidence of RCC has increased by 38% in the last two decades. This is in part the result of the increase in incidental detection resulting from the widespread use of ultrasound and CT scanning

- At the time of diagnosis, about 20% of patients have metastatic carcinoma and 25% have locally advanced disease

- Smoking, obesity, exposure to carcinogens (e.g. cadmium), and hypertension contribute to the development of RCC

- There is an increased incidence of RCC in patients with von Hippel–Lindau syndrome (VHL), horseshoe kidneys, adult polycystic disease, and acquired renal cystic disease from uraemia

- The link between VHL and RCC suggests a genetic predisposition

- RCC are vascular tumours which spread by direct invasion or along the renal vein or by lymphatic spread

Clinical presentation

- The majority of patients present with haematuria and loin pain – with or without a mass

- RCC is detected as an asymptomatic incidental lesion in at least 20% of cases. Ultrasound and CT scanning are the investigations that detect incidental RCC in the majority of cases

- Renal carcinoma may also present with a variety of paraneoplastic symptoms and pyrexia of unknown origin and for this reason it is known as the 'great imitator'

- A variety of haematological disorders may be seen, including anaemia from bleeding or marrow replacement, polycythaemia or thrombocytosis

- Performance status is the major predictor of prognosis and patients with poor performance status are unlikely to survive more than 2 years

Key Facts

Terms for RCC, such as hypernephroma, clear cell carcinoma, and alveolar carcinoma, have been used and reflect the historical controversy over the histogenesis of the disease.

Histologically most renal cell tumours are adenocarcinomas.

Treatment of localized RCC

- The mainstay of treatment of RCC is radical nephrectomy increasingly recently using laparascopic techniques

- Formal regional lymphadenectomy has not been shown to improve survival

- The presence of involved lymph nodes is a very poor prognostic indicator and is associated with a 5% 5-year survival

- Extension of the tumour into the inferior vena cava should be managed surgically by removal of the tumour embolus from the vena cava. Occasionally the thrombus will extend beyond the liver and into the right atrium. In such cases it is necessary to perform cardiac bypass surgery to enable excision of the thrombus

- Direct infiltration of the vena caval wall is associated with a poor prognosis

- There is currently no evidence that adjuvant treatment after radical nephrectomy improves prognosis. However, trials of immunotherapy are ongoing. For patients with good performance status and soft tissue metastases in whom immunotherapy is planned, nephrectomy may prolong survival. It should not be performed in patients whose performance status and prognosis are already poor, or if technically difficult. In such cases, symptomatic benefit, e.g. control of pain or bleeding, may be achieved by embolization of the blood supply to the tumour under radiological guidance. If metastases present late after nephrectomy, there is benefit from surgical excision of those metastases if they are solitary, or in the case of lung metastases only, even if multiple

Treatment of metastatic RCC

Some patients will present with a solitary metastatic lesion in the lung or brain. It is recommended that a nephrectomy be performed and 3 months after nephrectomy the patient should be re-evaluated. If there is still a solitary lesion, then metastases at these sites should be resected. This type of disease may be associated with long survival.

Prognosis in RCC

- The survival of patients with RCC is directly related to the extent of malignancy at the time of treatment

- Radical nephrectomy is curative in the majority of patients with localized disease; however, the risk of future relapse depends on the stage of the cancer at resection and the histological features

Future Possibilities

RCC exhibits multidrug resistance and at present no useful chemotherapy-only regimen exists for treatment. There have been sporadic reports of spontaneous regression of metastatic lesions in patients with RCC. This phenomenon is rare but suggests that RCC may be immunoresponsive. Presently interferon-alpha (IFN-α) and interleukin-2 (IL-2) are the two commonest forms of treatment for metastatic RCC. Side effects include fevers, chills, malaise. Nausea and vomiting are especially marked with IL-2. Recent evidence does suggest that IFN-α and IL-2 in combination with the chemotherapy agent 5-fluorouracil improve both progression-free interval and overall survival. The modest response rate and significant toxicity of immunotherapy mean it should be reserved for fit patients. New oral agents that target angiogenesis (e.g. sorafanib (a small-molecule tyrosine kinase inhibitor) and bevacizumab (the anti-vascular endothelial growth factor mono-clonal antibody)) have shown promising results in clinical trials and are entering clinical practice.

◆ Overall the prognosis for patients with metastatic disease is very poor and the 5-year survival for patients presenting with metastases is less than 15%

Cancer of the urothelium

Background

◆ Accounts for 1% of all cancers

◆ 90% are transitional cell cancers (TCC)

◆ 5–10% are squamous carcinoma

◆ 2% are adenocarcinoma

◆ 50–100 times more likely to occur in the bladder than other areas of urothelium

Risk factors for TCC include:

◆ Smoking

◆ Occupational exposure to aromatic amines and azo dyes

◆ Cyclophosphamide therapy

◆ Phenacetin-containing analgesics

Squamous cell carcinoma of the bladder is less common and associated with schistosomiasis, bladder calculi, or chronic irritation

---

Key Facts

TCC can be divided into: superficial bladder cancer and muscle invasive bladder cancer.

Superficial cancer (i.e. it has not breached the muscularis mucosa) is usually curable.

5-year survival of muscle invasive bladder cancer < 50%.

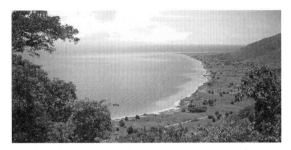

Fig. 13.5 Exotic travel to places like Lake Malawi exposes an international population to the local risks of schistosomiasis, including bladder squamous cell carcinoma.

Key Facts

The urothelium extends from the calyces of the kidney to the fossa navicularis of the penis in men and the proximal 50% of the urethra in women.

Presentation

◆ Painless haematuria 90% of cases

◆ Frequency

◆ Urgency

◆ Symptoms of metastatic disease

Diagnosis

Patients should have an abdominal ultrasound scan and cystoscopy as primary investigation of haematuria.

CT/MRI detects lymph nodes and metastatic disease in invasive bladder cancer.

Staging

This consists of:

◆ Careful bimanual examination prior to endoscopy

◆ Recording site and size of tumours

◆ Biopsy of tumours with samples from tumour base labelled

TABLE 13.3	Staging of bladder cancer
Stage	**Definition**
Superficial tumour	
Ta	Confined to mucosa
T1	Invasion into lamina propria
Tis	Carcinoma *in situ*
Invasive tumour	
T2a	Invasion of inner half of muscularis
T2b	Invades deep muscle (outer half)
T3a	Microscopic invasion of perivesical fat
T3b	Macroscopic invasion of perivesical fat
T4a	Invasion into prostate, uterus, or vagina
T4b	Invasion of pelvic or abdominal wall
Lymph node (N)	
N0	No regional lymph nodes
N1	Single regional lymph node < 2 cm
N2	Single regional lymph node > 2 cm < 5 cm
N3	Node > 5 cm
Distant metastasis (M)	
M0	No distant metastasis
M1	Distant metastasis

◆ Random samples of bladder and prostate urothelium looking for dysplastic changes

◆ Repeating bimanual examination following resection to assess if cystectomy is possible

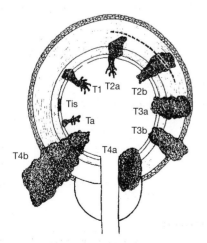

Fig. 13.6 TNM classification of bladder cancer. Tis = carcinoma *in situ*. Ta and T1 are classified as superficial.

Treatment

70–80% of all bladder cancers are 'superficial' – that is they do not invade the muscularis mucosa.

'Superficial' tumours

Treated with transurethral resection, many tumours will recur so follow-up with regular cystoscopy is mandatory.

Factors which identify patients likely to develop invasive disease and thus needing 3-monthly cystoscopy include:

◆ High-grade tumours

◆ Tumours which have breached the basement membrane

◆ Multiple tumours

Such patients may benefit from intravesical chemotherapy (Mitomycin C® or doxorubicin most commonly used). Evidence shows that such therapy prolongs disease-free interval and hence reduces the burden of cystoscopy surveillance.

Intravesical immunotherapy with BCG (Bacillus Calmette–Guèrin), a live attenuated vaccine, has been used to treat superficial bladder cancer by inducing a host immunological response. The risk is that occasionally patients can develop tuberculosis and require careful monitoring during treatment. BCG is the treatment of choice for bladder carcinoma *in situ* with complete responses in 50–70% of patients. High-grade T_1 disease is often treated with cystectomy if BCG fails to control the disease.

'Invasive' tumours

Disease which invades the muscularis mucosa of the bladder may be treated with radical cystectomy or radiotherapy. These modalities have not been directly compared and decisions regarding the choice of therapy tend to be based on performance status with surgery reserved for the younger and fitter patients. Bladder cancer is moderately chemosensitive. Neoadjuvant chemotherapy confers a 5% benefit in 5-year survival. Patients with locally advanced or metastatic disease may benefit from palliative chemotherapy. Active agents include cisplatin, gemcitabine and paclitaxel. No regimen is considered standard and these patients should be considered for entry into clinical trials.

Problems associated with progressive disease in cancer of the urothelium

◆ **Bladder spasm** can be frequent and troublesome leading to urinary frequency as well as pain

- **Pelvic pain** is common in advanced disease because of tumour progression. This pain can be extremely difficult to control as it is often complex and includes neuropathic elements. Anaesthetic interventions, including intrathecal and epidural procedures may be needed to gain pain control

- **Recurrent haematuria** is common and may be sufficient to cause anaemia and urinary retention as a result of clot retention. Catheter blockage may be a problem

- **Urinary incontinence** may occur

- **Urinary tract infections** as a result of long-term indwelling catheters are common but do not need treatment unless symptomatic

- **Lymphoedema** of the lower limbs and occasionally the genital area is usually the result of advanced pelvic disease. It needs to be actively managed by lymphoedema experts if the miserable effects of this symptom are to be minimized

- **Fistulae** may occur which are often suitable for surgery. If surgery is not possible the risks of skin breakdown are high

- **Renal failure** may occur. Stenting the renal tract may be possible but is not always appropriate and needs full discussion

- **Altered body image and problems with sexual function** are understandably common

- **Depression** is common because of the long course of the disease, sleep disturbance, and damage to self-esteem

Testicular cancer

Incidence and mortality

In 2001 1,996 men were diagnosed with testicular cancer in the UK.[5]

In 2003 89 men died from testicular cancer in the UK.[6]

- Testicular cancer represents approximately 1% of cancer in men but is important because even advanced disease can be cured

- 90–95% are germ cell tumours derived from the germinal epithelium of the testes

- Tumours are slightly more common on the right and are bilateral in 1–2% of cases

- The incidence of testicular carcinoma has doubled in the last 20 years but with the development

---

CLINICAL CASE

RB: TCC of the ureter

A 65-year-old man, RB, had presented with painless haematuria on three occasions in the past 3 months.

He had no other symptoms and no significant past medical history. He smoked heavily for 25 years, but had given up 5 years previously.

He had worked in a tyre factory for 15 years.

On examination RB was normotensive and full systems examination was unremarkable.

Investigation

Urinalysis revealed 3+ of blood. An intravenous pyelogram showed underfilling of the pelvis with a possible lesion in the pelvis of the kidney.

Endoscopy showed a normal lower urinary tract.

A CT scan demonstrated a mass in the renal pelvis on the left side.

A specimen of urine from the left kidney was obtained for cytology which showed malignant cells from a TCC.

Treatment

A nephro-ureterectomy with excision of a cuff of bladder was performed and the patient made an uncomplicated recovery. Histological examination of the specimen confirmed the presence of TCC with no invasion of the lamina propria.

Follow-up

Check cystoscopy 3 months later was normal and further follow-up with yearly cystoscopy was planned.

TABLE 13.4   Risk factors for testicular cancer

Recognized risk factors	
Cryptorchidism	Strongest risk factor (3–14-fold increase in risk) resulting in a 3–5% chance of developing cancer in either testis
Age	Seminoma occurs, on average, 10 years later than non-seminomatous germ cell tumours
Race	4 × incidence in white population compared with black

Implicated risk factors	
Genetic	Reported in siblings and twins but no definite association

of effective chemotherapy regimens, the overall 5-year survival is in the order of 90%

Clinical presentation

- Most commonly a painless unilateral swelling, usually found incidentally by patient or partner

- Scrotal pain occurs in up to one-third of patients

- 10% of patients present with acute testicular pain and 10% with symptoms from metastatic disease

- The contralateral testicle should be examined and biopsied if undescended or of small volume or if the patient is aged under 30 years

Investigations

- Clinical examination, including examination of the spermatic cord and scrotum

- Scrotal ultrasound to confirm the presence of a testicular mass

- All patients with testicular cancer should have tumour markers estimated preoperatively. These include α-fetoprotein, human chorionic gonadotrophin, and lactate dehydrogenase. Higher levels have an adverse prognosis

- A pre-operative chest X-ray and CT scan of chest, abdomen, and pelvis

TABLE 13.5   Tumour types in testicular cancer

Tumour type	(%)
Seminoma	40
Non-seminomatous germ cell tumours (NSGCT)	40
Teratoma differentiated	
Malignant teratoma intermediate	
Malignant teratoma undifferentiated	
Malignant teratoma trophoblastic	
Yolk sac tumour	
Mixed tumour (NSGCT and seminoma)	15
Other tumours	5
Stromal tumours	
Sertoli cell	
Leydig cell	
Lymphoma	
Leukaemia	
Carcinoma of the rete testis	
Metastatic	

TABLE 13.6   Summary of seminoma treatment

Stage	Treatment
I	Surveillance, chemotherapy and radiotherapy to para-aortic nodes
II A,B	Chemotherapy or radiotherapy to para-aortic nodes
II C onwards	Chemotherapy

Treatment of testicular cancer

Initial management of all patients:

- Inguinal orchidectomy with insertion of testicular prosthesis

- Completion of staging investigations

- Counselling regarding semen storage if further therapy required

Seminoma

Stage I (tumour confined to testis). Occult retroperitoneal nodal metastases in 15–20% of patients. Radiotherapy to these nodes (20 Gy in 10 fractions over 14 days) will result in 98% cure rate. One or two cycles of chemotherapy are also effective in stage I and may prevent the late effects of radiotherapy.

Stage II (enlarged retroperitoneal or pelvic lymph nodes). Radiotherapy to retroperitoneal and pelvic nodes (36 Gy in 18 fractions over $3\frac{1}{2}$ weeks) gives ≥ 95% cure rate. Again, two cycles of chemotherapy is an alternative. If lymph nodes are larger than 5 cm or cannot be treated with radiotherapy due to inclusion of kidney in the radiation field then treat with chemotherapy as for stage III

Stage III disease is treated with four cycles of cisplatin and etoposide and gives > 90% cure rate.

NSGCT

Stage I – If there is no lymphovascular invasion, and markers are normal, intensive follow-up (surveillance) with regular assessments of tumour markers and CT scans will result in 90% of patients remaining disease-free. Chemotherapy will salvage almost all patients who relapse on surveillance.

If pathology reveals lymphovascular invasion then risk of relapse is above 50%. Giving two cycles of chemotherapy with bleomycin, etoposide, and cisplatin (BEP) will cure 98% of these patients.

Stages **II/III/IV** – Cycles of BEP chemotherapy are given after assessment of prognosis. If residual masses remain in lungs or retroperitoneum after chemotherapy these should be resected by a specialist surgeon where possible. Approximately 40% of the resected masses will contain fibrotic tissue only, 40% will contain mature teratoma (with a risk of late relapse as a result of malignant change over many years if not resected), and 20% will have residual active tumour.

Even patients with the most adverse prognostic features have at least a 50% chance of cure.

References

1. http://info.cancerresearchuk.org/cancerstats/types/prostate/incidence/
2. http://info.cancerresearchuk.org/cancerstats/types/prostate/mortality/
3. http://info.cancerresearchuk.org/cancerstats/types/kidney/incidence/
4. http://info.cancerresearchuk.org/cancerstats/types/kidney/mortality/
5. http://info.cancerresearchuk.org/cancerstats/types/testis/incidence/
6. http://info.cancerresearchuk.org/cancerstats/types/testis/mortality/

Chapter summary

Prostate cancer

- Approximately 30% of all cancers in men
- The lifetime risk of developing prostate cancer is 30%; only 10% will be clinically significant
- The Gleason scoring system is based on the degree of glandular differentiation which is closely associated with disease progression
- Causes of an elevated PSA
  - Benign prostatic hyperplasia
  - Prostate cancer
  - Prostate infection
  - Prostate biopsy

Management

- Cancer confined to prostate gland
  - If aged < 70 and fit, give radical local therapy, e.g. prostatectomy, radiotherapy
  - If over 70 years 'Wait and see'
- Metastatic disease
  - Hormonal manipulation aimed at reducing the effect of androgens (mainly testosterone) at a cellular level will produce responses in around 70% of men with bone metastases with a median response duration of 12–18 months

Renal carcinoma

- Accounts for only 3% of all adult malignancies
- Risk factors: smoking, obesity, exposure to carcinogens (e.g. cadmium), and hypertension
- The mainstay of treatment of RCC is radical nephrectomy
- The 5-year survival for patients presenting with metastases is less than 15%

Cancer of the urothelium

- Accounts for 1% of all cancers
- TCC can be divided into superficial bladder cancer and muscle-invasive bladder cancer
- Superficial cancer is curable by transurethral resection and regular follow-up
- 'Invasive' tumours (5-year survival < 50%) treated by radical cystectomy or radiotherapy and palliative chemotherapy for metastatic disease

Testicular cancer

- Testicular cancer represents approximately 1% of cancer in men
- 40% seminomas, 40% non-seminoma germ cell tumours (NSGCT), 15% mixed
- Treatment of testicular cancer
  - Initial management of all patients – inguinal orchidectomy with insertion of testicular prosthesis, and completion of staging investigations
  - Radiotherapy and/or chemotherapy depending on stage of tumour give high cure rates
  - In selected patients, a retroperitoneal node resection is appropriate (done by a specialist)

CHAPTER 14

Patients with tumours of the central nervous system

'To expect a personality to survive the disintegration of the brain is like expecting a cricket club to survive when all of its members are dead.'
Bertrand Russell 1872–1970, British Philosopher, Mathematician, Essayist

Incidence and mortality

In 2001 2,550 men and 1,921 women were diagnosed with central nervous system (CNS) cancer in the UK.[1]

In 2003 1,946 men and 1,441 women died from CNS cancer in the UK.[2]

Background

♦ There are many tumours of the nervous system and there is still controversy over their classification

♦ Most brain tumours are metastatic from primary sites outside the CNS

♦ Primary brain tumours account for approximately 2% of all cancers

  • Primary brain tumours tend to remain localized to the CNS

  • Age: tumour incidence peaks in the 65–74 age group

  • Gender: men have a higher incidence

  • Race: incidence higher in white population than black in the USA

  • Social class: incidence higher in upper social classes

  • International variation is not very striking

  • No correlation proven to date with mobile phones

Gene disorders

TABLE 14.1 Neural tumours and gene disorders

Gene disorder	Tumour type
Neurofibromatosis type 1	Astrocytoma, optic glioma, neurofibroma
Neurofibromatosis type 2	Schwannoma, meningioma
Turcot syndrome	Glioblastoma, medulloblastoma
Tuberose sclerosis	Subependymal astrocytoma
von Hippel–Lindau syndrome	Haemangioblastoma
Gorlin syndrome	Medulloblastoma
Sturge–Weber disease	Choroid plexus papilloma

Gliomas

Gliomas (50% of all CNS tumours) comprise:

♦ **Astrocytomas** – account for 80% of gliomas, the most commonly occurring primary brain tumour; grade is important in determining prognosis

♦ **Oligodendrogliomas** – account for 10–15% of gliomas and commonly occur in the frontal lobes; longer prognosis

♦ **Ependymomas** – account for 5% of gliomas and tend to occur in children and young adults; may metastasize within the CNS

Other malignancies of the CNS

Pituitary adenomas (20% of all CNS tumours)

Treated medically for endocrine symptoms; treated surgically if there are pressure symptoms or visual field problems.

Meningiomas (25% of all CNS tumours)

Usually benign. Aetiological factors are previous radiation and trauma, particularly if it has led to chronic irritation.

> **Key Facts**
>
> The following characteristics are used to assess astrocytoma grade:
>
> ♦ Cell pleomorphism
>
> ♦ Mitotic activity
>
> ♦ Vascular proliferation
>
> ♦ Necrosis

Vascular (2% of all CNS tumours)

Angioma, haemangioblastoma.

Cerebral lymphoma (associated with immunosuppression)

1–2 per million per year, increasing in incidence partly as a result of HIV-associated malignancy.

Medulloblastoma

Accounts for 25% of all childhood tumours (cell of origin unknown). Maximal incidence at 3–5 years of age; 70% in children, 30% in adults; 70% of patients cured.

Spinal tumours

♦ Astrocytoma (may be high or low grade and have a variable prognosis)

♦ Ependymoma (can be the low-grade e.g. myxopapillary type or the intermediate to high-grade tumour of the cervico-thoracic cord in adults)

♦ Lymphoma (can very rarely occur as tumours within the cord – intramedullary – or more frequently as tumours compressing the cord – extradural)

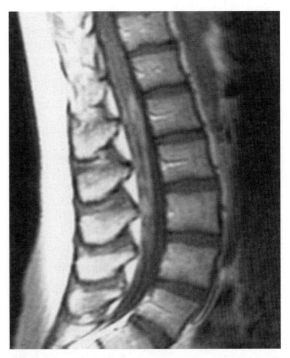

Fig. 14.1 Intramedullary lymphoma involving conus and cauda equina (very rare).

- Meningioma (resection can be difficult and prognosis depends on adequate resection)

- Chordoma (a tumour of notochord remnants occurring in the sacrum and clivus; surgery is the treatment of choice; radiotherapy may be required for significant residual disease or relapse)

- Schwannoma (this tumour of the peripheral nervous system can occur on spinal nerve roots and cause spinal cord compression)

- Neuroblastoma (this paediatric peripheral nervous system tumour can access the spinal canal through the intervertebral foramina, causing spinal cord compression)

Space-occupying lesions (SOL)

SOL is the term used when imaging of the brain shows a mass but as yet a pathological diagnosis has not been made. Imaging using computerized tomography (CT) scanning or magnetic resonance imaging (MRI) can give the following important information:

- Intra- versus extra-axial (within brain substance or outside)

- Contrast enhancement (how much intravenous contrast is taken up)

- Mass effect (how much compression of surrounding brain)

- Oedema (how much fluid is accumulated around tumour)

- Cysts (presence of abnormal fluid-filled cavities)

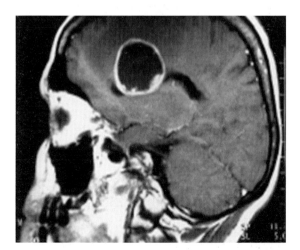

Fig. 14.2 SOL showing rim contrast enhancement. (CT scan with contrast.)

- Hydrocephalus (dilatation of ventricles caused by a block in cerebrospinal fluid (CSF) circulation)

An SOL can be caused by a cerebral abscess or cerebral bleed, as well as by cerebral tumours. The symptoms at presentation can be similar for all three conditions.

Symptoms

The presentation symptoms of brain tumours include:

- Raised intracranial pressure – headache (especially in the morning) and vomiting

- Epilepsy – petit mal, grand mal, temporal lobe type

- Neuropathies – hemiparesis, cranial nerve loss

- Posterior fossa signs – loss of balance/co-ordination

- Functional loss – personality change, cognitive loss, dysphasia

Investigations

- Contrast-enhanced CT scan

- Gadolinium-enhanced MRI scan

- Isotope scanning (position emission tomography, single photon emission computed tomography)

- If CSF spread is anticipated (e.g. for high-grade ependymoma) a neuroaxis MRI ± CSF for cytology is required after raised intracranial pressure has been excluded, i.e. no oedema/mass effect

- Biopsy is usually required to confirm diagnosis

Management of primary brain tumours

Surgery

Where it is possible, surgical resection alone for some low-grade tumours may be curative. Radiotherapy may be used as an alternative or adjunct to surgery.

For higher grade lesions, decompression of the tumour may provide palliation and facilitate post-operative radiotherapy. Radiotherapy may be given if surgery is incomplete depending on the site. Delayed radiotherapy is probably as effective as immediate radiotherapy in this situation. It has recently been shown that the addition of chemotherapy to radiotherapy has an advantage in some patients.

A decompressive operation leads to a pathological diagnosis, resolution of pressure symptoms, and improvement in function, allowing more patients to proceed with post-operative radiotherapy.

Radiotherapy

For high-grade gliomas, post-operative radiotherapy adds to the effectiveness of surgery and increases median survival from 5 to 11 months.

Not only can survival be improved, but for many there will also be significantly improved quality of life with adequate working abilities.

The ideal radiotherapy dose is 60 Gy but practically this can only be given to patients with good performance status.

For tumours with a propensity for leptomeningeal spread, such as high-grade ependymoma or medulloblastoma, cranio-spinal irradiation may improve prognosis.

Chemotherapy

Chemotherapy has a limited role to play in the treatment of most brain tumours and its use remains to be clearly defined. Some response to temozolamide can be expected or to the combination of procarbazine, CCNU, and vincristine (PCV) in recurrent disease. There is a role for temozolamide following local treatment of glioblastoma multiforme. Chemotherapy is also the principal treatment of CNS lymphoma and important as adjuvant therapy for medulloblastoma.

Prognosis

As a general rule in patients with brain tumours poorer prognosis is related to:

♦ High tumour grade

♦ Neurological deficit at presentation

♦ Older age at presentation

Key Fact

The most common brain tumour is a secondary lesion (brain metastasis)

This can present as single or multiple lesions and can arise from the following primary sites:

♦ Lung

♦ Breast

♦ Colorectal

♦ Skin – melanoma

♦ Testis

♦ Less commonly, oesophagus or stomach

Management of secondary brain tumours

Brain metastases

Autopsy reveals that metastases are commoner than revealed clinically: 60% of patients with small cell lung carcinoma and 75% with melanoma have brain metastases.

Carcinoma of the prostate, bladder, and ovary *rarely* metastasize to the brain.

The prognosis for brain metastases is dependent on the primary cancer, the performance status at presentation, and the response to treatment.

Assessment

Clinical history

♦ Neurological examination of higher cortical function, cranial nerves, musculoskeletal system, sensation, cerebellar function, and gait

Clinical features

Symptoms and signs can evolve over days to weeks. Multiple deposits are present in over two-thirds of patients and clinical signs depend on the anatomical site.

♦ Focal neurological disturbance consists of motor weakness including hemiparesis (30%), dysphasia, and cranial nerve palsies

♦ Epileptic seizures (15–20%)

♦ Raised intracranial pressure, e.g. especially morning headache (50%), nausea, vomiting, and lethargy

♦ Change in mood, cognitive function or behaviour

Investigations

CT or MRI scan (more sensitive, especially for tumours situated in the posterior fossa or brainstem) show the location of metastases, surrounding oedema, and mass effect.

Management

Radical treatment

Surgery may be suitable for a small percentage of patients who are young, fit, and have only a solitary metastasis and this disease is not progressing elsewhere. Suitability for surgery also depends on the anatomical site of the tumour.

Patients who might benefit from aggressive management of brain metastases include those with chemosensitive tumours such as the haematological malignancies, small cell lung cancer, and possibly breast cancer.

Palliative treatment

Initial corticosteroids and palliative radiotherapy are usually the most appropriate treatments and may improve neurological symptoms and function in over 70% (with a median survival of 5–6 months). This enables a gentle reduction and sometimes withdrawal of steroids after 4–6 weeks following treatment.

Cranial irradiation

Benefit may not be gained in those patients with poor prognostic factors which include poor performance status, age over 60 years, non-breast primary site, multiple lobe involvement, short disease-free interval, and overt uncontrolled metastases elsewhere.

Decisions regarding treatment should be, as ever, tailored to the problems of the individual patient.

Cranial irradiation may cause some degree of scalp or upper pinna erythema and irritation.

Alopecia is universal in this population. Unfortunately prognosis is unlikely to allow regrowth of hair within the remaining lifespan.

The start of treatment may induce an increase in cerebral oedema which may require readjustment of the steroid dose.

Other effects of cranial radiotherapy include transient somnolence, occurring within a few weeks, and longer term impairment of memory and cognition. These are significant problems in very few people and most patients do not survive long enough for late radiation changes in the CNS to develop.

In patients who have a chemosensitive primary tumour (e.g. breast or small-cell lung cancer) and extracranial disease as well as cerebral metastases, chemotherapy may be considered as an alternative to cranial irradiation.

Corticosteroids

High-dose corticosteroids (dexamethasone 16 mg/day initially) reduce cerebral oedema, and associated symptoms of headache and vomiting may be helped rapidly.

In certain situations, particularly with tumours in the posterior fossa, hydrocephalus may be present, in which case a ventricular shunt may be required for symptom control.

The short prognosis for most patients means that the issue of long-term side effects of steroids may not be a problem. It is best practice, however, to gradually reduce the dose to the lowest possible over a few weeks to minimize potential side effects since difficulties may build up insidiously.

A stage may be reached when the dose necessary to control the cerebral oedema causes significant side effects.

Disabling problems such as obesity (and associated problems with immobility), body image problems, proximal myopathy, mood swings, fragile skin, and diabetes may then develop. There should be open dialogue (particularly while the patient is alert and can join in discussions) about the ongoing use of steroids in the event that quality of life becomes adversely affected.

Patients and families may view the steroids as agents to control the disease and resist attempts to reduce the dose, fearing the return of symptoms of raised intracranial pressure.

On the other hand, patients may have recognized that their quality of life is deteriorating despite continuing steroids and may then agree to their withdrawal. This should generally be done slowly while controlling the symptoms of raised intracranial pressure by other means.

When patients become moribund and can no longer swallow, steroids can generally be stopped but this may depend on the particular clinical circumstances and may need negotiation with the patient/family. There should be adequate medication provision (subcutaneous) for analgesia, anti-emetics, anticonvulsants, and sedatives as necessary.

Stop and Think

Multiple complex physical and psychological problems including poor mobility, complex care needs, swings in mood, uncertainty in prognostication, and confusion can completely exhaust even the most caring family, who need the expert support of an experienced multidisciplinary team.

Prognosis

It is very difficult to predict prognosis accurately in patients with brain tumours.

Although some patients, particularly with metastases from breast cancer, may survive relatively longer, most patients with brain metastases from solid tumours have a survival of a few weeks or months at best.

Metastatic disease of the leptomeninges (meningeal carcinomatosis)

Five per cent of patients with tumours may develop clinical signs and symptoms of leptomeningeal disease although the rate at autopsy is higher (10%). It is most commonly seen in lymphoma and leukaemia although it may occur in breast cancer, small cell lung cancer, and melanoma.

Clinical features

The presenting features may be varied and fluctuating and the diagnosis should be considered in any unexplained neurological disturbance in a patient with cancer. The most frequently encountered are cranial nerve problems (75%), headache (50%), radicular or back pain (40–45%), and weakness in one or more limbs (40%). Other presentations include meningism, altered consciousness, confusion, sphincter disturbance, and seizures. Abnormal physical signs are more prominent than symptoms, with lower motor neurone lesions predominating.

Investigations

♦ **Lumbar puncture** if there is no evidence of raised intracranial pressure (90% will have positive cytology and increased protein on CNS analysis)

♦ **MRI scan** to look for enhanced meningeal signal

Management

This may include intrathecal chemotherapy, depending on the tumour type. Radiotherapy has limited and only short duration benefit. The aim is to halt progression of disease and relieve symptoms but it is essentially pallia-

---

CASE HISTORY

RJ: Cerebral lymphoma

A 59-year-old man, RJ, presented with headache, ataxia, and then collapse. CT scan showed a lesion in the right parietal lobe of the brain (Fig 14.3).

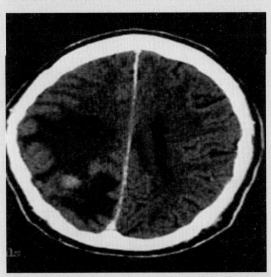

Fig. 14.3 CNS lymphoma in a periventricular location.

Decompression was performed and histology showed a high-grade B-cell non-Hodgkin's lymphoma. Staging was by MRI scan of craniospinal axis (clear), CSF cytology (clear), and CT scan of thorax, abdomen, and pelvis (clear).

His primary treatment was a chemotherapy regimen containing high-dose methotrexate and cytarabine with folinic acid rescue. Sodium bicarbonate diuresis was required to facilitate methotrexate clearance.

RJ's first course of chemotherapy was complicated by an episode of thrombocytopenia 10 days into the cycle, requiring platelet transfusion.

During the second course of chemotherapy, the methotrexate was not cleared through his urine in 2–3 days despite optimal diuresis, contributing to a drop in haemaglobin.

The development of anaemia caused conversion of his controlled atrial fibrillation to uncontrolled atrial fibrillation.

Blood transfusion and folic acid supplementation stabilized his condition.

Imaging showed complete response to chemotherapy. He then proceeded to cranial radiotherapy. He received a dose of 30 Gy in 15 fractions over 3 weeks. The fields included posterior orbit and cribriform plate (sanctuary sites for relapse). He has remained disease free for 1 year.

Lessons

♦ Lymphoma can appear similar to glioma on imaging

♦ Optimal chemotherapy regimens can be toxic despite precautions

♦ Serum methotrexate levels must be measured to determine when adequate clearance has been achieved

♦ High-dose whole brain radiotherapy can cause cognitive function loss

♦ Results are reasonable for reduced dose radiotherapy, especially if complete response is achieved with chemotherapy

♦ To reduce the risk of a demyelinating encephalopathy, high-dose chemotherapy should be given first in sequence before radiotherapy, although the combination in any order is still a risk factor for demyelination

tive except for a curable sub-group with leukaemia or lymphoma. Steroids and non-steroidal anti-inflammatory drugs may help symptoms.

Prognosis

Without treatment, patients may survive for several months depending on the tumour type with relentless progression of neurological symptoms. Even with treatment, prognosis is usually less than 6 months and is worst in small cell lung cancer, widespread disease, patients with poor performance status, and where there are widespread neurological signs.

References

1. http://info.cancerresearchuk.org/cancerstats/types/brain/incidence/
2. http://info.cancerresearchuk.org/cancerstats/types/brain/mortality/

Chapter summary

Background:
- Most brain tumours are metastatic from primary sites outside the CNS
- Primary brain tumours account for approximately 2% of all cancers
- Age: adult primary brain tumour incidence peaks in the 65–74-year age group

Primary brain tumours include:
- Gliomas (50% of all CNS tumours)
- Pituitary adenomas (20% of all CNS tumours), treated medically for endocrine symptoms
- Meningiomas (25% of all CNS tumours)

Treatment:
- Surgical resection for some low-grade tumours may be curative
- For high-grade gliomas post-operative radiotherapy prolongs the effectiveness of surgery
- Chemotherapy has a limited role to play in the treatment of most brain tumours

Secondary brain tumours:
- The most common brain tumour is a secondary lesion (brain metastasis)
- These can present as single or multiple lesions and classically arise from the following primary sites:
  - Lung
  - Breast
  - Colorectal
  - Oesophagus or stomach
  - Skin – melanoma
- Symptoms and signs can evolve over days to weeks
- Multiple deposits are present in over two-thirds of patients
- Surgery is suitable for a small percentage of fit, young patients with no disease elsewhere
- Initial corticosteroids and palliative radiotherapy are the commonest treatments
- Most patients with brain metastases from solid tumours have a survival of a few weeks or months

CHAPTER 15

Patients with common haematological malignancies

Chapter contents

Background

* The malignant haematological conditions considered individually are relatively uncommon but:

  * Acute lymphoblastic leukaemia (ALL) is the commonest cancer of childhood

  * Taken together, the haematological malignancies are the most common cause of cancer in the working population

* The haematological malignant cell populations result from clonal proliferation by successive divisions from a single transformed stem cell

* In most haematological disorders, there is a slight male preponderance

* The definitive diagnosis of these conditions requires cytochemical, immunocytochemical, cytogenetic, and, occasionally, molecular techniques

* Balancing opportunities for cure with impact of treatment on life quality are crucial in assessing the appropriateness of interventions which by their nature are often extremely aggressive and taxing for patients

* Chemotherapy has led to marked improvements in survival over the last 40 years

Simple definitions

* Leukaemia – cancer of the blood-forming cells of the bone marrow

* Lymphoma – cancer of the various cells of the lymph glands

* Myeloma – cancer of the plasma cells of the bone marrow

* Myelodysplastic syndromes (MDS) – malformation of the haemopoietic cells frequently progressing to acute leukaemia

* Myeloproliferative disorders – low-grade malignancy of multipotent bone marrow precursor cells

---

Key Fact

A simple classification of leukaemia:
Acute myeloblastic – AML
Acute lymphoblastic – ALL
Chronic myeloid – CML
Chronic lymphocytic – CLL

Stop and Think

Leukaemia is by its nature widespread at the time of diagnosis and almost any organ may be involved. These problems require close cooperation between haematologists, nephrologists, intensive-care specialists etc.

Leukaemia

Incidence and mortality

In 2001 3,833 men and 2,922 women were diagnosed with leukaemia in the UK.[1]

In 2003 2,453 men and 1,886 women died from leukaemia in the UK.[2]

Aetiology

The majority of cases of leukaemia have no recognizable aetiological factors though a long list of factors has been suggested.

Pathology

Leukaemias may be subdivided into acute and chronic, myeloid and lymphatic

The **acute leukaemias** are characterized by the accumulation of blast (*primitive*) cells in the bone marrow. These cells are usually also present in the peripheral blood, sometimes in high numbers. Acute leukaemia is characterized by a rapid cellular proliferation and a corresponding rapid disease course. The patient may quickly develop life-threatening complications such as neutropenic sepsis unless treated promptly.

The **chronic leukaemias** are characterized by the accumulation of cells that have differentiated *beyond the blast stage*. Organ dysfunction may develop after many months/years because of the accumulation of malignant cells.

Chronic lymphocytic leukaemia (CLL) presents with mature lymphocytes in excessive numbers in both peripheral blood and bone marrow.

In **chronic myeloid leukaemia** (CML) there is an excessive production of cells of the myeloid line from blast cells through to mature granulocytes, although an increase in the relative proportion of primitive precursors is not uncommon.

Presentation

Patients with leukaemia are likely to present with one of three groups of symptoms:

- Anaemia
- Infection
- Bleeding

Examination

Clinical examination may reveal the features of anaemia, infection, or bleeding.

Purpura may be widespread or localized and should be sought on the hard or soft palate or the retina.

Fifty per cent of patients with ALL, and even more with chronic lymphatic leukaemia, will have lymphadenopathy though this is rare in myeloid leukaemias.

Patients with CML may present with 'massive splenomegaly' while those with CLL are more likely to present with widespread lymphadenopathy.

Diagnosis and staging

Peripheral blood count and examination of a blood film are essential.

Although there is frequently anaemia and thrombocytopenia, the white cell count may be normal, low, or raised.

Examination of the peripheral blood film will usually demonstrate the presence of abnormal cells. Confirmation of the diagnosis is made by examining a bone marrow smear and performing appropriate cytochemical, immunocytochemical, and cytogenetic examinations. Flow cytometry is now an essential part of the diagnostic work-up in acute and chronic leukaemias.

Key Facts

Bone marrow investigation

- Samples are usually taken from the posterior iliac crest, using local anaesthetic (short-acting benzodiazepine may also be used)
- It is usual to take a core of bone (trephine biopsy) in addition to aspirating marrow
- The trephine biopsy is particularly useful in those cases where there is a dry tap (no marrow can be sucked out) or a blood tap (what is sucked out is the same as blood)
- Patients with low platelets may rarely require platelet transfusion to prevent excessive bruising and bleeding from the procedure

---

Key Facts

Acute emergency in AML

- Of particular importance is the **acute** promyelocytic leukaemia variant (APML)
- APML almost always involves a chromosomal translocation t(15:17) that results in the fusion of the retinoic acid receptor alpha (*RAR alpha*) gene with a transcription factor gene called *PML*
- Patients with this condition comprise one of the most acute medical emergencies as the granules in the promyelocytes release thromboplastin, causing disseminated intravascular coagulation which can lead to life-threatening haemorrhage. However all-*trans* retinoic acid, has proved very effective in reducing diffuse intravascular coagulation in this condition

---

As leukaemia is normally widespread at the time of diagnosis, staging is usually inappropriate; chronic lymphocytic leukaemia is an exception.

Acute myeloblastic (myeloid) leukaemia (AML)

Morphological, cytochemical, and immunocytochemical examination of the blood and marrow from patients with acute myeloid leukaemia (AML) allows categorization depending on the presence, to a greater or lesser degree, of myeloid, monocytic, erythroid, or megakaryocytic features.

Cytogenetics

The strongest prognostic factor in AML is cytogenetics. Balanced translocations [t(8;21), t(15;17) and inv16] confer a good prognosis and complex karyotypes confer a poor prognosis.

Treatment

The most effective treatment for AML consists of a combination of an anthracycline, e.g. daunorubicin and cytarabine.

Depending on age and cytogenetics, up to 80% of patients will achieve remission, with younger patients faring better.

For young patients with unfavourable characteristics at diagnosis (high white cell count and adverse chromosomal abnormalities), bone marrow transplantation from a human leucocyte antigen (HLA)- matched sibling is the treatment of choice, giving cure rates as high as 50%.

Similar regimens may be tried in older patients but concomitant disease and frailty, together with more common adverse chromosomal abnormalities, mean that treatment is much less frequently successful.

In the very old patient there is an argument in favour of supportive treatment only, particularly when the white cell count is not high, as median survival is in the order of only 6–8 weeks.

Prognosis

The advent of modern chemotherapeutic techniques and supportive therapies has improved the prognosis for patients with AML from 6 weeks to many months/years for the responsive patient.

Quality of life

Successful treatment of acute leukaemia is highly specialized as patients may be extremely susceptible to infection, bleeding, and many other complications.

Prompt and vigorous management of complications can best be undertaken in specialist units.

Improved prognosis in these patients is not only the result of new treatments but also of better support and aggressive symptom management.

In the initial stages, which require prolonged periods of hospitalization, the patient may be severely tested physically and emotionally.

Acute lymphoblastic leukaemia (ALL)

- ALL is the common form of leukaemia in children and has an age peak under 5 years of age
- Immunophenotyping has shown that ALL may be of either B- or T-cell precursor types
- 'Common' ALL, a subtype of B-lymphoblastic leukaemia, accounts for the majority of cases
- Central nervous system (CNS) leukaemia is common in patients with ALL and cerebrospinal fluid should be examined at an early stage to exclude this possibility

Key Facts

Favourable prognostic features in ALL

- Young (but not < 2 years)
- Female
- White race
- 'Common' type
- No CNS disease at presentation
- < 4 weeks to achieve remission

Treatment

- Although the combination of prednisone and vincristine can induce remissions in up to 90%, long-term survival is markedly improved with the addition of more drugs in the induction period
- Remission induction is therefore nearly as aggressive as in AML, although the remission rate, particularly in children, is higher
- Because of the frequency of meningeal leukaemia (up to 75% of cases not given prophylaxis), 'prophylactic' treatment begins after the first consolidation therapy and consists of high-dose intravenous methotrexate or cranial irradiation and intrathecal methotrexate
- Patients normally receive up to 6 months of intensive therapy (including cranial prophylaxis) before progressing to maintenance therapy
- Maintenance therapy usually consists of continuous mercaptopurine, weekly methotrexate (both oral), and monthly intravenous injections of vincristine with short courses of prednisolone
- Such therapy yields 'cure' rates of 75–80% in children under 16
- The cure rate drops rapidly with age. In the older age group, consideration must therefore be given to bone marrow transplantation, whereas in children, transplantation is normally only used after relapse occurs and a second remission has been induced

Prognosis

- In patients with good prognosis, long-term survival rates are in excess of 80% with rates falling as adverse factors accumulate
- Patients achieving long-term remission can lead normal lives
- CNS irradiation affects some aspects of intelligence, particularly in the very young, and for this reason it is normally delayed until the patient is at least 2 years old or high-dose methotrexate is used instead
- Isolated relapses in sanctuary sites, e.g. testes, may be treated by local radiotherapy before or after further induction and maintenance therapy, sometimes followed by local radiotherapy

Quality of life

- The majority of children cope well with the side effects and complications of treatment during the induction, consolidation, and maintenance phases

- They will be relatively susceptible to infection and appropriate measures such as administration of vaccine immune globulin must be taken if they encounter viral infections such as chickenpox

- In older patients quality of life is largely determined by remission duration

Chronic myeloid leukaemia (CML)

- CML is characterized by a raised white cell count and the presence in the peripheral blood of all stages of immature cells, from blast cells to mature granulocytes

- There is frequently splenic enlargement

- The platelet count may be elevated and the patient is usually anaemic

- The vast majority of cases of CML possess the Philadelphia chromosome t(9;22), producing the fusion gene *bcr-abl*

- CML may also first present in its transformed state (blastic transformation)

Treatment

- Although CML will respond to a wide variety of cytotoxic agents, it remains an essentially incurable disease unless treated with an allogeneic stem cell transplant

- The oral agent hydroxyurea reduces the white cell count and improves symptoms but Philadelphia-positive cells remain, indicating persistence of the malignant clone. Hydroxyurea has fewer long-term side effects than busulphan, which is equally effective but is associated with drug-related acute leukaemia

- Interferon by contrast requires subcutaneous injection and produces Philadelphia-negative haemopoiesis in a proportion of patients. Side effects, e.g. flu-like symptoms, are common

- The tyrosine kinase inhibitor, imatinib mesylate, which is targeted against the effect of the Philadelphia chromosomal translocation, is highly effective and has produced a major change in the treatment of CML. A high proportion of patients achieve Philadelphia-negative haemopoiesis

- Prior to the use of imatinib, patients up to the age of 50–55 years were given cytoreductive therapy with hydroxyurea, followed by allogeneic transplantation from a sibling donor whenever available. Such patients are now treated with imatinib and transplantation is reserved for non-responding patients

- If no sibling donor is available, bone marrow registers should be searched for an unrelated matched donor in patients up to the age of 30

Prognosis

- Any form of treatment which reduces the leucocyte count and the size of the spleen will produce clinical benefit

- Patients may develop 'accelerated disease', when they become relatively resistant to treatment with conventional agents, or 'blastic transformation', where there is a progression to an acute leukaemia (usually myeloid) with chromosomal changes

- The response to intensive chemotherapy is generally poor. Median survival for chronic-phase patients without allogeneic transplantation used to be in the order of 4 years but this is improving with the use of imatinib

Quality of life

- Simple drug treatment significantly improves quality of life and overall survival. Imatinib offers improved response and tolerability compared to previous treatments such as interferon

- Bone marrow transplantation may offer improved survival (even 'cure') but is a high-risk procedure with significant side effects such as graft-versus-host disease (GvHD)

- Patients receiving long-term interferon may experience significant side effects

Chronic lymphocytic leukaemia (CLL)

CLL is a relatively indolent disease, mainly of the elderly; some patients may never require treatment.

CLL is confirmed using immunophenotypic methods to differentiate the condition from other lymphoproliferative disorders, some of which are associated with an adverse prognosis compared to 'classical' CLL.

Binet staging system

TABLE 15.1 Binet staging system CLL

Stage	Gland/organ enlargement	Haemoglobin (g/dl)	Platelets (×10⁹/l)
A	0, 1, or 2 areas	≥ 10	≥ 100
B	3, 4, or 5	≥ 10	≥ 100
C	Not considered	< 10	<100

Treatment

Asymptomatic stage A patients do not require treatment.

Patients with stage B or C disease may need treatment, particularly if there is evidence of bone marrow failure, symptomatic involvement of lymph nodes, splenomegaly, or systemic symptoms such as weight loss or excessive sweating.

Symptoms and signs of autoimmune haemolytic anaemia and/or thrombocytopenia are common in CLL and are a further indication for treatment.

Patients with bone marrow failure or autoimmune haemolytic anaemia/thrombocytopenia should receive corticosteroids prior to the commencement of chemotherapy.

For other patients, alkylating agents such as chlorambucil are the usual initial therapy and may be combined with corticosteroids. Patients becoming resistant to these agents may be treated with newer drugs such as fludarabine, alone or in combination chemotherapy, e.g. CHOP (see section on non-Hodgkin's lymphoma, page 140).

Recent evidence suggests improved response, and possibly survival, with fludarabine-based combination therapy. Addition of the anti-CD20 monoclonal antibody rituximab has had an impact on response and promises much for future improvement in response rates.

Radiotherapy is useful for treatment of areas of bulky disease, including lymph nodes and/or spleen. Patients with CLL have impairment of the immune system and will require active antibiotic treatment for infections and possibly prophylaxis with antibacterial, antifungal, or antiviral drugs.

Younger patients may be suitable for allogeneic stem cell transplantation, which offers the prospect of cure but also the risk of serious toxicity as previously discussed.

Prognosis

'Classic' CLL presenting in the elderly, especially when it is found from a routine blood count rather than as the result of symptoms, may not require immediate therapy or indeed any therapy at all.

Patients may continue to lead a relatively normal life and some may never require treatment.

In younger patients or in those with more advanced disease, i.e. stage B/C, treatment will be required and median survival is significantly reduced compared to age-matched controls.

If remission can be induced, prognosis is significantly improved.

Long-term cure is unlikely without allogeneic transplantation.

Quality of life

For indolent disease presenting in the elderly, quality of life may be little affected.

Younger patients or those with more aggressive disease are likely to require intensive therapy, affecting quality of life as well as survival.

Lymphoma

The lymphomas are a group of tumours caused by primary malignancy of lymphoid cells.

Their wide diversity reflects the complexity of these organs.

They are normally considered in two major groups:

◆ Hodgkin's disease

◆ Non-Hodgkin's lymphomas

Lymphoma accounts for approximately 4% of all cancers.

They occur with a relatively high frequency in young adults.

They are treatable and in some instances curable.

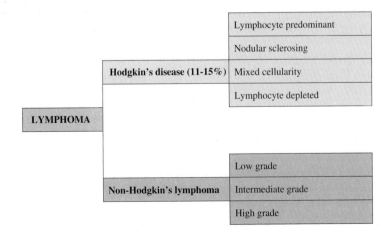

Fig. 15.1 Classification of lymphomas.

Hodgkin's disease

Incidence and mortality

In 2001 814 men and 612 women were diagnosed with Hodgkin's lymphoma in the UK.[3]

In 2003 175 men and 135 women died from Hodgkin's lymphoma in the UK.[4]

Background

- Hodgkin's disease is a group of related disorders sharing some common pathological features and clinical behaviour

- The disease is named after Thomas Hodgkin who described the first cases at Guy's Hospital in 1832

- Hodgkin's disease has a bimodal age distribution with the first peak occurring in young adults between the ages of 15 and 34 and the second peak in older patients

- A number of factors point to a possible aetiology involving the Epstein–Barr virus in at least some cases of Hodgkin's disease

- In some studies, a seasonal incidence has been shown

- No preventative measures or screening techniques have been developed

Presentation

- Patients may present with isolated or multiple swellings of lymph nodes or symptoms arising from enlargement of the lymph nodes, i.e. enlargement of the nodes of the mediastinum may cause obstruction to the return of blood from the head and upper limbs: superior vena cava syndrome

- Other manifestations include generalized symptoms such as weakness, lassitude, loss of appetite, weight loss, abnormal sweating (particularly at night) which may be severe, itch, and very occasionally pain at nodal sites on ingestion of alcohol

- Where Hodgkin's disease is suspected, palpation of neck, axilla, and groins is especially important. Mediastinal involvement may be suspected on chest examination, and abdominal palpation may reveal an abdominal mass or enlargement of spleen and/or liver

Diagnosis

Lymph node biopsy is necessary for diagnosis.

Pathology

The nature of the malignant cell in Hodgkin's disease has been the subject of debate for many years, though it is now believed that the Reed–Sternberg cell is the primary tumour cell and is of B-cell origin.

Reed–Sternberg cells constitute a minority of abnormal cells within a background of reactive cells including lymphocytes, plasma cells, and eosinophils.

In some instances, bands of fibrous tissue are seen (nodular sclerosing variant).

Staging

TABLE 15.2	Ann Arbor staging system (simplified)
Stage	
I	Involvement of single lymph node region or lymphoid structure (e.g. spleen, Waldeyer's ring)
II	Involvement of two or more lymph node regions or structures on same side of the diaphragm
III	Involvement of lymph node structures or regions on both sides of the diaphragm
IV	Involvement of extranodal site(s), e.g. liver, bone marrow
A	No symptoms
B	Fever, drenching sweats, weight loss (> 10% in 6 months)
E	Involvement of a single extranodal site

- Clinical staging is of importance with regard to both prognosis and choice of treatment

- The Ann Arbor scheme was devised in the 1960s and is universally accepted

- Staging requires not only careful clinical examination but chest X-ray, computerized tomographic (CT) scan of chest, abdomen, and pelvis, and preferably one more imaging technique for abdominal glands such as ultrasound or gallium scanning

Treatment

- Stages IA and IIA disease are suitable for treatment with short-course chemotherapy, often followed by involved field low-dose radiotherapy. If patients are staged correctly, this will be curative in approximately 90% of cases

---

Key Facts

Hodgkin's disease and constitutional symptoms

The presence or absence of constitutional symptoms (B symptoms) is of great significance.

B symptoms are defined as weight loss equal to or greater than 10% of total body weight in the past 6 months, significant night sweats – usually sufficient to require the patient to change night clothes/sheets – or unexplained fever of > 38°C.

♦ Patients relapsing after radiotherapy may be 'salvaged' by chemotherapy

♦ Patients with more advanced disease, i.e. stages III and IV and all patients with B symptoms, should receive chemotherapy

♦ The four-drug regimen devised by Vincent de Vita in the late 1950s, known as **MOPP** and consisting of mustine, Oncovin® (vincristine), procarbazine, and prednisone given in short courses followed by time for marrow recovery, represented one of the great strides forward in the treatment of malignant disease, with more than 50% of patients with advanced disease being cured of their illness. New regimens have displaced MOPP, e.g. ABVD (Adriamycin®, bleomycin, vinblastine, dacarbazine) constitutes the current 'gold standard' because it has equivalent outcome but reduced adverse effects such as infertility or second tumours. Five-year survival is about 80%, with most patients achieving long-term cure

♦ Patients relapsing after conventional chemotherapy may achieve second remissions with the same drugs, but remission duration is usually shorter than the previous remission

♦ However, high-dose therapy with autologous peripheral blood or bone marrow transplantation gives high remission rates in relapsed patients and long-term disease-free survival in the order of 50%

Prognosis

Defective immune function may remain in patients with Hodgkin's disease for many years and patients should be warned to be on their guard for infections from serious and opportunist pathogens.

Late relapse following therapy may occur, though the majority of patients who are disease-free 5 years following the cessation of treatment are cured.

Long-term sequelae include increased risk of malignant disease, including therapy-related acute myeloid leukaemia, lung and other solid malignancies. In recent years, women who have had mantle radiotherapy for lymphoma while young have required mammographic screening in later life.

Patients with hyposplenism or who have had the spleen removed are at risk from septicaemia, particularly with encapsulated organisms such as *Pneumococcus*, *Meningococcus*, and *Haemophilus* species.

Quality of life

Most of the above chemotherapy regimens can be given on a day-patient/outpatient basis.

Side effects have been reduced with modern antiemetics and leucopenia is only rarely of sufficient severity to require inpatient treatment for sepsis, etc.

With ABVD-type therapy, gonadal function may be retained and for many patients there are few long-term sequelae.

Non-Hodgkin's lymphoma (NHL)

Incidence and mortality

In 2001 4,910 men and 4,371 women were diagnosed with non-Hodgkin's lymphoma (NHL) in the UK.[5]

In 2003 2,472 men and 2,202 women died from NHL in the UK.[6]

♦ The histopathological classification of NHL is complicated

♦ The WHO scheme for classifying NHL has gained most acceptance

♦ This scheme makes use of morphological appearance, immunocytochemical, cytogenetic, and molecular data to identify meaningful subgroups which are of prognostic significance

♦ It is helpful to consider NHL in broad categories, depending on clinical behaviour, which may be rapid and highly aggressive (commonly described as high grade) or indolent and slowly progressive (commonly described as low grade)

♦ **Low-grade lymphomas** run a chronic course, frequently respond to simple chemotherapy, and may have remissions lasting from a month to many years, but most will eventually relapse with progressive disease. No significant cure rate has been as yet achieved

♦ **Intermediate- and high-grade lymphomas** run a more aggressive course and some high-grade lymphomas are potentially rapidly fatal. A significant

TABLE 15.3 Predisposing diseases in NHL	

Immune dysfunction
  AIDS
  Inherited
  Therapeutic immunosuppression,
  e.g. chemotherapy, radiotherapy
	Usually B-cell high or intermediate grade

Coeliac disease Dermatitis herpetiformis Angioimmunoblastic lymphadenopathy	Usually T-cell lymphomas
Intestinal infections Autoimmune diseases, e.g. rheumatoid arthritis, systemic lupus erythematosus	Marginal zone B-cell lymphoma

proportion will respond to multidrug chemotherapy and enduring remissions are possible for a proportion of patients

- Although the frequency of NHL is increasing, aetiology remains uncertain. Various predisposing conditions have been identified, including immunodeficiency, HIV infection and Epstein–Barrvirus

Pathogenesis

- Enlargement of lymph nodes is a predominant feature of NHL
- The disease is presumed to arise in one site, although it is frequently widely disseminated by the time diagnosis is made
- The superficial glands are often involved but involvement of nodes of the mediastinum/abdomen or pelvis without superficial lymphadenopathy is not uncommon
- Bone marrow involvement may lead to anaemia, leucopenia/neutropenia, or thrombocytopenia
- The gastrointestinal tract is the most commonly involved extranodal site after bone marrow
- Other organs such as skin, brain, testes, or thyroid may be involved and CNS lymphoma is relatively frequent in AIDS patients

Diagnosis and staging

- Presentation will depend on the nodes and other organs involved
- Constitutional symptoms such as fever, night sweats, and weight loss occur less frequently than in Hodgkin's disease and usually indicate disseminated disease
- Lymph node biopsy is usually required for diagnosis
- The Ann Arbor staging scheme is generally applicable to NHL
- NHL is more frequently widely disseminated at diagnosis than Hodgkin's disease
- Bone marrow aspirate and trephine biopsy are required for the exclusion of marrow disease
- A CT scan should be used to show the presence or absence of intra-abdominal involvement

Treatment

- Treatment varies significantly with the type of lymphoma diagnosed

- Low grade:
  - Anti-CD20 monoclonal antibody (rituximab) is effective in treatment of B-cell lymphoma, either alone or in combination with chemotherapy
  - Low-grade lymphoma may be treated with relatively non-aggressive therapy delivered as an outpatient as severe reduction of the white cell and platelet counts is unlikely

- High grade:
  - For intermediate and high-grade lymphoma, the CHOP regimen (intravenous cyclophosphamide, doxorubicin, vincristine and oral prednisolone) remains the gold standard treatment
  - More intensive regimens have failed to improve on long-term survival rates of properly administered CHOP
  - Addition of anti-CD20 monoclonal antibody to CHOP appears to improve the response rate and survival in B-cell lymphomas
  - The role of high-dose therapy with bone marrow or peripheral stem cell rescue is still being evaluated but has the potential to achieve long-term remission in relapsed patients with high-grade lymphoma

Prognosis

- Prognosis varies greatly depending on the precise diagnosis
- Low-grade lymphoma runs an indolent course – in some patients repeated remissions can be obtained with relatively simple therapy and a proportion of patients may live for 15 or 20 years, although cure is unlikely
- Intermediate and high-grade lymphoma behaves in a more aggressive fashion and response to simple single-agent chemotherapy is poor
- More intensive chemotherapy such as the CHOP regimen produces long-term disease survival in 30–50% of patients
- Prognosis is adversely affected by disease subgroup, patient age (older than 60–65 years), poor performance status, multiple sites of extranodal disease, etc

Myeloma

Incidence and mortality

In 2001 1,928 men and 1,640 women were diagnosed with multiple myeloma in the UK.[7]

In 2003 1,332 men and 1,291 women died from multiple myeloma in the UK.[8]

Background

+ Myeloma (also called multiple myeloma or myelomatosis) is a neoplastic monoclonal proliferation of bone marrow plasma cells

+ The aetiology of myeloma is unknown

+ The disease may typically affect bone, kidneys, and the immune system

+ Curative treatment remains elusive

+ The disease affects older patients, reaching a peak in the seventh decade

+ The disease is characterized by increased numbers of plasma cells in the bone marrow. The condition is therefore widespread at diagnosis but marrow involvement may be patchy

+ Occasionally a single lesion may be present – this is known as a plasmacytoma and may later lead to widespread disease

+ The course of the disease is related to the presence in the bone marrow of malignant plasma cells and the distant effect of their products

+ Plasma cells are responsible for immunoglobulin production

+ In myeloma the plasma cells may secrete a single monoclonal immunoglobulin (M-protein), either on its own or with the additional excretion of light chains. The M in this instance refers to the *monoclonal* nature of the protein and not the immunoglobulin subclass which may be IgG, A, M, D, or E

+ ESR often grossly elevated

+ In about 15% of cases this paraprotein is absent, with production of light chains only, which are excreted in the urine, known as Bence-Jones proteinuria

+ Immunoglobulin light chains may precipitate in the renal tubules, leading to renal failure, which is associated with poor survival

+ Myeloma cells may also secrete a number of cytokines which have local and distant effects, contributing significantly to the production of lytic bony lesions

+ Very rarely, the malignant plasma cells do not produce abnormal immunoglobulin (non-secretory myeloma) and patients thus exhibit features of bone marrow replacement without a detectable paraprotein

Presentation

Clinical findings relate to the effect of the myeloma cells and their products on other organs.

Key Facts
Relative frequency of M-proteins
IgG 56%
IgA 27%
IgM < 1%
IgD 1%
IgE rare
Light chain only 15%
Non-secretory 1%
(No M protein production)

Lytic bone lesions may cause pain, e.g. in the back, and are usually visible on plain X-ray. Plasma protein electrophoresis and a urine sample for Bence-Jones protein should be part of the investigation of any patient aged over 40 with persistent back pain.

Hypercalcaemia may lead to polydipsia, polyuria, anorexia, vomiting, constipation, and mental disturbances.

Bone marrow replacement by malignant plasma cells may lead to anaemia and repeated infections, which are usually related to deficient antibody production, although in advanced disease neutropenia may also be present.

TABLE 15.4 How malignant plasma cells may affect other organs

Organ	Effect of myeloma	End result
Bones	Local expansion with bone destruction (aided by cytokine excretion)	Lytic lesions Pathological fractures Collapsed vertebrae Hypercalcaemia
Kidney	Light chain deposition in tubules	Renal failure
Bone marrow	Marrow replacement	Anaemia, etc.
Immune system	Suppression of normal immunoglobulin production	Immunosuppression infections
Blood	Excess protein	Hyperviscosity
Other organs	Amyloid deposition Local invasion Non-metastatic distant effects	Dysfunction Neuropathy, etc.

Renal impairment is frequent and multifactorial because of the effects of the paraprotein or light chain on the kidney, hypercalcaemia, dehydration, side effects of analgesic drugs, e.g. non-steroidal anti-inflammatory drugs, or infection.

Non-metastatic distant effects of myeloma

♦ Myeloma may produce a hyperviscosity syndrome because of the very high immunoglobulin levels. Effects include reduced flow in small blood vessels, with CNS features ranging from altered vision to confusion and reduced consciousness in the most severely affected. Abnormal platelet function and bleeding may occur

♦ Features of amyloid deposition may develop, such as macroglossia, carpal tunnel syndrome, diarrhoea, or cardiac dysfunction

♦ Laboratory findings include:

  • Raised erythrocyte sedimentation rate, raised total protein (except in Bence-Jones and non-secretory myeloma), abnormal protein electrophoresis, and reduced immunoglobulin levels

  • Anaemia is frequent

  • Hypercalcaemia may occur on its own or with raised urea and creatinine, indicating renal failure

Diagnosis

Diagnosis usually requires a demonstration of two key features.

Particularly in non-secretory myeloma, the diagnosis may be made on the bone marrow appearances only.

Key Facts

Key features in diagnosing myeloma

1. Excess monoclonal plasma cells usually > 30% in bone marrow
Note: trephine biopsy may be more accurate than aspirate

2. Significant monoclonal paraproteinaemia and/or Bence-Jones proteinuria

3. Radiological evidence of lytic lesions (osteoporosis is non-specific)

Staging

TABLE 15.5 Myeloma may be staged into groups I, II, or III according to the Salmon–Durie staging system.

Stage	
I	All of
	♦ Hb > 10 g/dl
	♦ Normal serum calcium
	♦ No X-ray lytic lesions (or solitary plasmacytoma only)
	♦ Low M-protein production rates
	(a) IgG < 50 g/l
	(b) IgA < 30 g/l
	(c) Urinary light chain excretion < 4 g/24 hours
II	Fitting neither stage I nor III
III	One or more of the following:
	♦ Hb < 8.5 g/dl
	♦ Raised serum calcium
	♦ Advanced lytic bone lesions
	(a) IgG > 70 g/l
	(b) IgA > 50 g/l
	(c) Urinary light chain excretion > 12 g/24 hours
A	Relatively normal renal function
B	Abnormal renal function

Treatment

Multiple myeloma is incurable by conventional means although there is a possibility of cure with allogeneic transplantation. Unfortunately the presenting age/fitness of most patients rules out this mode of therapy.

The introduction of oral melphalan and prednisone 40 years ago offered control of symptoms and significantly improved survival from a few months in untreated patients to several years in those responding. Progress since has been slow and various melphalan-based regimens were not found to improve outcome. However, multi-agent chemotherapy e.g. VAD (vincristine, Adriamycin®, dexamethasone) followed by autologous stem cell transplantation has been shown to prolong survival significantly. The novel proteosome inhibitor, bortezomib, can control relapsed disease for a time. Local bone symptoms can be controlled using local radiotherapy.

Prognosis

Median survival is 30–36 months.

Patients presenting with advanced disease (particularly renal failure) have a much worse prognosis.

Future Possibilities

Recently thalidomide and its analogues have been shown to be effective and relatively non-toxic. Mode of action may include alteration of the cytokine environment of the myeloma cell. Promising responses have also been noted with bortezomib, a novel agent that inhibits the proteasome (the cellular machinery that breaks down peptides).

Stop and Think

Quality of life

Patients with newly diagnosed myeloma are usually treated as outpatients and may maintain a reasonable quality of life. However, bony involvement and chronic pain are common and often require the help of a palliative care or pain management specialist in symptom management.

Related conditions – other causes of paraproteins

An abnormal paraprotein may be found in other haematological conditions.

Monoclonal gammopathy of uncertain significance (MGUS)

MGUS is associated with the presence of an M-protein. However, the low level of production, the small size of the implicated paraprotein, the absence of lytic lesions, and insufficient plasma cells in the marrow preclude the diagnosis of myeloma. The M-protein level may remain unchanged for many years or slowly progress to frank myeloma.

An IgM paraprotein may be associated with a type of low-grade lymphoma with features of plasma cell differentiation (lymphoplasmacytoid) known as Waldenström's macroglobulinaemia. Hyperviscosity may be a prominent feature as a result of the tendency of IgM to polymerize.

Other types of B-cell lymphoproliferative disease may be associated with an abnormal paraprotein, including chronic lymphatic leukaemia and hairy cell leukaemia.

Myeloproliferative disorders

Background

- The myeloproliferative disorders are a group of conditions characterized by proliferation of one or more of the haemopoietic components of the bone marrow; this group includes CML

- The conditions may evolve into each other, such evolutions generally signifying a worsening of prognosis

- Polycythaemia vera, essential thrombocythaemia, and myelofibrosis are considered as the non-leukaemic myeloproliferative disorders

- Myeloproliferative conditions are more common in the elderly

- Spleen and liver are frequently enlarged in these conditions

- Patients may present with features specific to the disease, e.g. plethora due to high haemoglobin in polycythaemia vera or massive splenomegaly in myelofibrosis

- Patients may also present with non-specific constitutional symptoms including lethargy, weakness, and weight loss

Primary proliferative polycythaemia (PPP)

Polycythaemia (also called erythrocytosis) is defined as a sustained increase in the haemoglobin and a subsequent rise in the haematocrit (> 0.52 in adult men and > 0.48 in women for longer than 2 months). There are many causes of polycythaemia – see box.

- It is a condition in which the increase in red blood cells is caused by endogenous myeloproliferation

- There is frequently an increase in granulocytes and platelets, indicating the stem cell nature of the disorder

- The clinical features are related to the overproduction of cells with resulting increase in blood viscosity, blood volume, and metabolic activity

- The *JAK2* mutation has been described in over 90% of patients with PPP

- **Clinical features of polycythaemia vera**

  - General – headaches, pruritis (especially after hot baths), dyspnoea, blurred vision, night sweats

  - Plethoric appearance – ruddy cyanosis, conjunctival suffusion, retinal venous engorgement

  - Splenomegaly (two-thirds of patients)

  - Haemorrhage (gastrointestinal, uterine, cerebral)

  - Thrombosis, arterial or venous

  - Hypertension (one-third of patients)

  - Gout (due to raised uric acid production)

  - Peptic ulceration (5–10% of patients)

Treatment

- The object of treatment is to maintain the blood count, particularly haemoglobin and red cell volume, within normal limits
- Where thrombocytosis also features, the platelet count should also be kept within normal limits and the patient should be given aspirin
- When the haemoglobin and platelet count are maintained at these levels there is a significant reduction in symptoms and complications, and long-term survival is possible
- The treatment of choice is therefore venesection
- Newly diagnosed cases with very high haemoglobin and haematocrit represent a medical emergency because of the risk of thrombosis
- Daily or alternate-day venesection may be used until the haemoglobin approaches normal levels, with subsequent venesection to maintain haemocrit < 0.45 (level at which adverse events unlikely)
- Control of the platelet count may require use of myelosuppressive agents. Polycythaemia vera is associated with an inherent risk of leukaemic transformation and this is increased by certain therapeutic agents with leukaemogenic effects. Most patients are treated with oral hydroxycarbamide (hydroxyurea) which is thought to have a very low risk of leukaemogenesis

Prognosis

- Once the haematocrit and platelet count are controlled the risk of complications (which are similar to the presenting features) is greatly reduced
- Many patients with polycythaemia vera may have a relatively normal lifespan; however, the risk of transformation to myelofibrosis or acute leukaemia is always present and will clearly modify the prognosis

Quality of life

- Whilst the condition remains as simple polycythaemia vera, and serious complications such as thrombosis are reduced by venesection, the quality of life is largely related to the degree of itch experienced by the patient. This is often aggravated by exposure to water (aquagenic)
- Control of itch may be very difficult but antihistamines or myelosuppressive therapies may be helpful. Some patients may require skin cleansing with baby oil or other means of avoiding water

Thrombosis and haemorrhagic complications affect both prognosis and quality of life.

Essential thrombocythaemia (ET)

Essential thrombocythaemia (ET) is a rare condition characterized by persistent overproduction of platelets. Platelet count at diagnosis may exceed $1,000 \times 10^9/l$ with associated megakaryocytic proliferation in the marrow. For diagnosis it is necessary to show a persistently elevated platelet count ($> 600 \times 10^9/l$) in the absence of any of the known causes of thrombocytosis.

Treatment

The optimal treatment for ET remains to be established but usually consists of a myelosuppressive agent such as hydroxyurea. Interferon may also be used and may carry a lower risk of leukaemic transformation. Alkylating agents, e.g. busulphan or radioisotope therapy with P[32] are less favoured because they carry a higher risk of leukaemic transformation.

Prognosis

Essential thrombocythaemia is a chronic condition providing death does not occur as a result of bleeding or thrombotic events.

Transformation may occur after a number of years to polycythaemia vera, myelofibrosis, or acute leukaemia.

Myelofibrosis

Background

- Myelofibrosis is characterized by replacement of the marrow by varying degrees of fibrosis associated with circulating primitive cells. Blood film findings include the presence of immature myeloid and nucleated erythroid cells (leucoerythroblastic) and alteration of red cell shape with frequent teardrop-shaped cells (poikilocytosis)

- Marrow fibrosis is thought to be the result of platelet-derived growth factors produced by the excessive number of megakaryocytes and in some instances the disease will develop from polycythaemia vera or essential thrombocythaemia

- Splenomegaly is frequent and may be massive, causing local discomfort and splenic pooling of red cells and platelets with resulting low counts

- Constitutional symptoms may also occur e.g. sweating, weight loss

- Early disease is often associated with anaemia caused by marrow dysfunction and splenomegaly, but a raised leucocyte and platelet count. Thrombocytopenia and leucopenia occur in later stage disease as the marrow reserve declines and splenic pooling worsens

- The current treatment options for myelofibrosis are unsatisfactory and do not appear to alter the progression of the condition. Symptomatic anaemia requires regular red cell transfusion and patients should receive folic acid supplementation. Hydroxycarbamide may be required for the control of leucocyte or platelet count and may improve constitutional symptoms

- Splenectomy may alleviate symptoms and reduce transfusion requirements, but is relatively high risk with significant postoperative mortality and morbidity

- Progression to acute leukaemia is not uncommon

Prognosis and quality of life

As patients tend to have progressive disease, life expectancy is poorer than for the other non-leukaemic myeloproliferative disorders. Correspondingly, quality of life tends to be more adversely affected because of the splenomegaly, anaemia, and requirement for blood transfusion.

Myelodysplastic syndromes (myelodysplasia; MDS)

Background

This is a group of clonal neoplastic disorders, producing qualitative and quantitative changes in the cells of the bone marrow and peripheral blood and with a tendency to progress to acute leukaemia. The bone marrow is often hypercellular and exhibits abnormal cell differentiation with a varying increase in blast cells. The WHO classification has replaced earlier schemes and has helped to identify factors with prognostic significance.

Aetiology is unclear but may be similar to that of acute leukaemia. Therapy-related myelodysplasia may occur some years after treatment with certain drugs, e.g. alkylating agents such as busulphan. Such cases have poor prognosis and a high rate of leukaemic transformation.

In general, there is inadequate production of one or more cell lines (red cells, white cells, platelets) and clinical problems may arise from anaemia, thrombocytopenia, or neutropenia/infection. Treatment tends to be largely supportive with red blood cell transfusion given as necessary although erythropoietin reduces red cell transfusion requirements and granulocyte colony-stimulating factor can improve leucocyte count and reduce infections. Regular platelet transfusion may be required.

Progression to acute leukaemia may occur rapidly or after years but is associated with poor prognosis and reduced chemotherapy response compared with *de novo* acute leukaemia.

There may be a role for bone marrow transplantation depending on age group and the availability of a matched donor.

Quality of life

Patients may live relatively normal lives for many years even if they remain transfusion dependent. Development of acute leukaemia is associated with an abruptly reduced quality of life.

Bone marrow support

The dose-limiting factor with most forms of chemotherapy is the ability of the marrow cells to recover their function before the patient dies through lack of immune defence mechanisms.

Short periods of profound neutropenia can usually be managed by means of vigorous treatment of infection with broad-spectrum antibiotics, antifungals, and antiviral agents as appropriate, together with intravenous fluids and resuscitation.

A number of mechanisms are available to augment the host defence in this situation:

- **Transfusion of neutrophils** – although their short half-life means that they are of limited benefit
- **Granulocyte and granulocyte–macrophage colony-stimulating factors** may be given to speed neutrophil recovery after conventional chemotherapy, and are effective in allowing modest increments in the dose of chemotherapy, or reduction in time between courses of chemotherapy. They are, however, less effective in patients given very high doses of chemotherapy (and do not avoid other side effects, e.g. stomatitis, diarrhoea)

The alternative approach is to provide the patient with a new source of **haemopoietic stem cells** following the delivery of high-dose chemotherapy.

Bone marrow transplantation

Stem cells may be obtained from the bone marrow by a harvest procedure under general anaesthetic and be stored during high-dose chemotherapy, then reinfused via a vein. This allows the stem cells that were not exposed to the conditioning regimen (high-dose chemotherapy or total body irradiation) to generate new blood cells, speeding the recovery of the blood count. There is, nevertheless, a period of several days with profound myelosuppression and risk of serious infection. Allogeneic transplantation carries specific additional risks. Transplants that use the patient's own stem cells (autografts) are more straightforward than those from a matched donor (allografts).

These relate to the development of GvHD (damage to the recipient by the donor immune system – unwanted and associated with adverse effects) and graft-versus-leukaemia effect (GvL – desired and associated with reduced relapse).

Key Facts

Types of stem cell transplant

- Allogeneic – stem cells obtained from a compatible donor
- Syngeneic – stem cells obtained from an identical twin
- Autologous – stem cells obtained from patients themselves (usually cryopreserved until required for transplant)

Graft-versus-host disease (GvHD)

- This may occur even in apparently perfectly HLA-, B-, and HLA-DR-matched sibling allogeneic transplantation
- The development is variable and relates to undiscovered tissue compatibility systems or minor variations in the identified systems
- *Acute* GvHD is characterized principally by skin rash, intractable diarrhoea, and abnormal liver function, and occurs in the first 100 days post-transplant
- *Chronic* GvHD occurs after 100 days
- Immunosuppressive agents are routinely used to try to prevent GvHD although a minor degree of GvHD (i.e. insufficient to cause serious morbidity) can be associated with an effect on the leukaemia or lymphoma (so-called graft versus lymphoma/leukaemia, or GvL, effect)
- GvHD is a potentially fatal condition; it also predisposes patients to opportunistic infections as do the agents used to suppress it
- These problems bring about a significant death rate in the period immediately following transplantation; despite this, long-term results are superior to conventional treatment for leukaemia and lymphoma in a number of situations
- Separation of the GvHD and GvL effects would allow enhanced tumour control without undesirable morbidity but has not been satisfactorily achieved

Stem cell transplantation

Peripheral blood stem cell transplantation is gaining in popularity over bone marrow transplantation because of the shorter time to recovery of neutrophil and platelet numbers following transplantation.

In this procedure, stem cells are obtained from the peripheral blood by a technique known as leucophoresis. Stem cells are normally present in the blood in very small numbers but numbers are dramatically increased using growth factors, and in the case of autologous donors, in the recovery period after chemotherapy.

Stem cells may also be obtained from the umbilical cord after delivery of the fetus, but umbilical cord blood transplants are only suitable for patients under 60 kg because of the limited numbers of stem cells normally available in cord blood donations. The longer time from transplantation to cellular recovery makes this form of treatment more difficult.

The stem cells, like a bone marrow transplant from whatever source, are given back to the patient by infusion into a vein following the completion of chemotherapy after enough time has been allowed for the drugs to be cleared from the system.

The stem cells find their own way to the bone marrow microenvironment where they proliferate to form blood cells.

Stop and Think

Patients with blood malignancies can face a particularly challenging treatment journey because the clinical course tends to be very variable, and is characterized by protracted cycles of relapse and remission.

- Patients with acute leukaemia do not generally spend a long time in the terminal stage unlike patients with myeloma
- The emotional component of having an 'incurable' disease is a huge issue for some patients and their families
- The age and impact of blood malignancies in children creates particular issues for families and staff

These points can create tensions between 'treatment centred' and 'symptom control centred' approaches.

- Identification of the terminal phase in haematology patients is very difficult
- Some patients with advanced haematological malignancy who are on the brink of death have been returned to an active normal life through aggressive therapy
- Conversely some patients who are still receiving active therapy die undergoing treatment with an emotive impact on the quality of their death
- After many months of treatment and patient–staff 'bonding', both the patient and the professionals may find it hard to acknowledge that the terminal phase is approaching

Symptomatic management of patients with advanced disease

Specific pain complexes in patients with haematological malignancies

- **Bone pain** is common in patients with myeloma. The pain is often worse on movement or weight-bearing which makes titration of analgesics very difficult. The pain often responds well to radiotherapy and/or oral steroids. Non-steroidal anti-inflammatory drugs may help but must be used with caution because they may interfere with platelet and renal function in patients who are often already markedly compromised in this regard

- **Pathological fractures** are particularly common in myeloma due to the lytic bone lesions. These often require orthopaedic intervention and subsequent radiotherapy. Prophylactic pinning of long bones and/or radiotherapy should be considered to prevent fracture and reduce the likelihood of complex pain syndromes developing

- **Spinal cord compression** requires prompt diagnosis, high-dose oral steroids in a single daily dose and urgent therapy to reduce compression, e.g. radiotherapy or surgical decompression. The steroids should be continued at a high dose until a definitive plan has been made. They may then be titrated down in accordance with the patient's condition and symptoms

- **Wedge and crush fractures of the spinal column** can lead to severe back pain which is often associated with nerve compression and neuropathic pain. Such pain is partially opioid-sensitive but adjuvant analgesics in the form of anti-depressants and/or anti-convulsant medication are usually required to supplement the effect of the opioid. Specialist advice is frequently needed to maintain symptom control

Other complications

- **Oral mucositis** is common with some chemotherapy regimens and can lead to severe reduction of oral intake. Opioid therapy via syringe driver is often required for this type of severe oral pain

- **Recurrent infections and bleeding episodes** can leave patients and carers exhausted

- **Night sweats and fever** are common, imposing a heavy demand on carers, particularly as several changes of night and bed clothes may be needed. Specialist advice may help in relieving the symptoms, as there are a number of drugs that can be tried

- **Hypercalcaemia** may occur, especially in myeloma. It should be considered in any patient with persistent nausea, altered mood or confusion (even if this is intermittent), worsening pain and/or constipation.

Treatment is with intravenous hydration and bisphosphonates. Resistant hypercalcaemia may be a pre-terminal event when aggressive management would be inappropriate.

CASE HISTORY

Mr H: Lymphadenopathy

'Dear Doctor,
This young man is unwell and has glands in his neck. Please advise…'

History

Mr H is aged 35 years and has been unwell for the past 3 months with loss of appetite, weight loss of 1 stone and night sweats, for which he has to change his night clothes usually once per night. For the past 2–3 weeks he has been short of breath and has poor exercise tolerance.

On examination he had multiple hard enlarged lymph nodes on both sides of the neck, axillae, and groins. Spleen and liver were not palpable and other systems were unremarkable.

Investigations

* Haemoglobin 12.1 g/dl
* Leucocytes 15.9 × 10⁹/l
* Platelets 460 × 10⁹/l
* Erythrocyte sedimentation rate 6 mm in the first hour
* Lactate dehydrogenase 1024 (N = 360–720)
* Remainder of the biochemical screening within normal limits
* Chest X-ray showed significant widening of the mediastinum
* CT scan showed enlargement of mediastinal, para-aortic, and iliac nodes
* Cervical lymph node biopsy showed Hodgkin's disease (nodular sclerosing, type II)

Treatment

Patient received six courses of ABVD (Adriamycin®, bleomycin, vinblastine, and dacarbazine).

Physical examination showed resolution of all palpable nodal enlargement and a complete response was confirmed by CT scan.

Chapter summary

* The malignant haematological conditions considered individually are relatively uncommon
* The definitive diagnosis of these conditions requires cytochemical, immunocytochemical, cytogenetic, and occasionally molecular techniques
* The **acute leukaemias** are associated with the accumulation of blast (*primitive*) cells in the bone marrow
* The **chronic leukaemias** are associated with the accumulation of cells that have differentiated *beyond the blast stage*

Acute myeloblastic leukaemia (AML)

* Morphological, cytochemical, and immunocytochemical examination allows categorization into one of eight subgroups
* Chemo- and supportive therapy have improved prognosis from 6 weeks untreated to many months/years in responsive patients
* 50–80% of patients will achieve remission, with younger patients faring better

Acute lymphoblastic leukaemia (ALL)

* ALL is the most common form of leukaemia in children
* Meningeal leukaemia may be present at diagnosis and will develop in up to 75% of cases not given prophylaxis
* Treatment is capable of achieving 'cure' rates of 75–80% in children under the age of 16
* The cure rate drops rapidly with age
* Patients receive up to 6 months of intensive therapy (including the cranial prophylaxis) before progressing to maintenance therapy

Chronic myeloid leukaemia (CML)

* The vast majority of cases of CML possess the Philadelphia chromosome t(9;22)
* It is an essentially incurable disease unless the patient receives an allogeneic transplant
* Treatment which reduces leucocyte count and spleen size will produce clinical benefit
* Median survival for chronic-phase patients is in the order of 4 years

Chapter summary—*cont'd.*

Chronic lymphocytic leukaemia (CLL)

- CLL is an indolent disease mainly of the elderly

- Some patients may never require treatment

- CLL may respond to single agent therapy, e.g. chlorambucil but enhanced response is seen with multi-agent therapy. Younger patients are usually treated more aggressively

- If remission can be induced, prognosis is significantly improved

- Except for patients who have successful bone marrow transplants, long-term cures are rare

Hodgkin's disease

- Lymph node biopsy is necessary for diagnosis

- Clinical staging is of importance with regard to both prognosis and choice of treatment

- Multi-agent chemotherapy given in short courses followed by time for marrow recovery can produce cure for up to 80% of patients

- Patients relapsing after conventional chemotherapy may achieve second remission and cure with autologous transplantation

Non-Hodgkin's lymphoma (NHL)

- The histopathological classification of NHL is complicated with many subtypes

- **Low-grade lymphomas** run a chronic course, often responding to simple chemotherapy

- **Intermediate and high-grade lymphomas** are more aggressive

- CHOP combined with a monoclonal antibody to CD20 (rituximab) offers enhanced response and survival compared to CHOP alone in aggressive B-cell lymphomas

- Prognosis is adversely affected by subgroup, patient age (> 60–65 years), poor performance status, and multiple sites of extranodal disease

Myeloma

- Predominantly a disease of older patients

- Malignant plasma cells secrete a single monoclonal, immunoglobulin (M-protein)

- Clinical findings relate to the effect of the myeloma cells and paraprotein on other organs

- Unless allogeneic bone marrow transplantation is possible myeloma remains incurable

- Median survival is 30–36 months

Myeloproliferative disorders

- Proliferation of one or more of the haemopoietic components of the bone marrow

- Myeloproliferative conditions are more common in the elderly

- Spleen and liver are frequently enlarged in these conditions

- *Polycythaemia vera* – increase in red blood cells by endogenous myeloproliferation

- *Essential thrombocythaemia* is a rare persistent over-production of platelets

- *Myelofibrosis* is characterized by marrow fibrosis associated with circulating primitive cells

References

1. http://info.cancerresearchuk.org/cancerstats/types/leukaemia/incidence/
2. http://info.cancerresearchuk.org/cancerstats/types/leukaemia/mortality/
3. http://info.cancerresearchuk.org/cancerstats/types/hodgkinslymphoma/incidence/
4. http://info.cancerresearchuk.org/cancerstats/types/hodgkinslymphoma/mortality/
5. http://info.cancerresearchuk.org/cancerstats/types/nhl/incidence/
6. http://info.cancerresearchuk.org/cancerstats/types/nhl/mortality/
7. http://info.cancerresearchuk.org/cancerstats/types/multiplemyeloma/incidence/
8. http://info.cancerresearchuk.org/cancerstats/types/multiplemyeloma/mortality/

Patients with skin cancers

Background

- Skin cancer is the most common cancer diagnosed in the UK as well as many other countries
- There are over 40,000 new cases of skin cancer annually in the UK – 90% are non-melanomatous
- The numbers of skin tumours increase steadily with age
- Ozone layer erosion has allowed a significant increase in the amount of ultraviolet (UV) light reaching exposed skin
- In the UK there is an annual 3% increase in rates of melanoma
- Most of the common cancers of the skin, apart from melanoma, are easily treated and the death rate is low compared to that for other solid tumours
- For this reason, skin cancers are often excluded in solid cancer 'league' tables

TABLE 16.1	Cell types in the skin
Epidermis	
Squamous	
Basal	
Melanocytes	
Langerhans – immunological	
Merkel – mechanoreceptors, APUD system	
Dermis	
Connective tissue – blood vessels, lymphatics, nerve supply	
Appendages – hair follicles, sebaceous and exocrine glands	

Key Facts

Causes of skin cancer

- UV light
- Genetic
- Atrophic skin lesions
- Chemical carcinogenesis
- Radiation exposure
- Immunosuppression

Aetiology of skin tumours

Ultraviolet (UV) light and the ozone layer

The UVB spectrum (290–320 nm) is the major carcinogenic wavelength. Basal cell carcinomas (BCC), in particular, but also squamous cell carcinomas (SCC), are more prevalent on light-exposed areas of the body, especially the dorsum of the hands and the face. Areas of vitiligo (depigmentation) lead to increased susceptibility.

Stop and Think

Global warming and skin cancer?
Normally the ozone layer in the stratosphere absorbs UVB from sunlight. Fluorinated hydrocarbons have reduced the thickness of the ozone layer, allowing more UVB to pierce the lower layers of the stratosphere. How much has the increase in skin cancer been the result of the destruction of the ozone layer?

Atrophic skin lesions

Skin cancer can result from skin damage which leads to atrophic lesions. It may also arise in chronic ulceration – breakdown of the epithelium in a recurring cycle of repair and ulceration.

Radiation exposure

In the past, radiotherapy was used to treat benign conditions such as acne and tinea capitis. Later it was found that there was an increased incidence of skin cancer in the treated areas.

Immunosuppression

Immunosuppressive drugs used to prevent rejection of transplants causes a striking increase in the incidence of all types of skin tumour.

HIV infection has produced a rise in Kaposi's sarcoma.

Stop and Think

Chemical carcinogenesis
In 1775, Sir Percival Pott described the first occupational skin cancer, that of the scrotal skin in boy chimney sweeps. The cancer was later shown to be the result of coal tar irritation of the scrotal folds.

Diagnosis

A full general examination of the skin in good light should be carried out, with a meticulous examination of each particular lesion together with the associated regional lymph node drainage areas.

Benign lesions

Seborrhoeic keratosis

- These are common and increase in incidence with age
- They are brownish lesions, round to oval in shape, with a slightly irregular non-shiny surface and a 'waxy or greasy' quality
- They can usually be treated with liquid nitrogen
- Alternatively, curettage may be used with light cautery to achieve haemostasis

Warts

These are common, viral-induced lesions that often resolve spontaneously. Occasionally biopsy may be required for definitive diagnosis. If persistent, they are treated with liquid nitrogen, though a number of applications may be necessary to achieve success.

Keratoacanthoma

This is a hyperkeratotic tumour, which clinically resembles a squamous cell carcinoma. It usually arises on sun-exposed skin in the central face but may also be seen on the dorsum of the hands and forearms. It is characteristically dome-shaped with a central plug of keratin. It usually has a short history of 2–4 weeks and tends to involute spontaneously over the next 4–5 months, often leaving a scar. These features distinguish it from squamous carcinoma, which has a longer history. If there is doubt, a wedge biopsy may be necessary.

Pre-malignant lesions

Solar (actinic or senile) keratosis

UVB damages the keratinocytes leading to multiple, red, rough papules of 1–3 mm in diameter. They tend to arise on sun-exposed areas, especially on the dorsum of the hand, face, neck, and nose. Over a long time they may progress to squamous cell carcinoma.

Heaped up lesions require a biopsy but otherwise a watching policy is reasonable.

Malignant lesions

The two most common lesions are basal cell carcinoma and squamous cell carcinoma. Of these, basal cell is the commonest.

Basal cell carcinoma (BCC)

This starts as a painless translucent pearly nodule with telangiectasia on a sun-exposed area. It grows slowly with local invasion over many years. As it enlarges, it ulcerates, bleeds, and develops a rolled, shiny border. For these reasons, it is often termed a rodent ulcer. Fortunately, metastases are rare. The face is the commonest site, and it rarely spreads to adjacent lymph nodes.

Squamous cell carcinoma (SCC)

These are red, irregular, hyperkeratotic tumours that ulcerate late and develop a crust. They generally occur on sun-exposed areas of the head and neck and dorsal extremities. Metastases to local lymph nodes occur more commonly than in basal cell carcinoma – amounting to 1–2% of cases. Challengingly, such tumours may also be associated with superficial infection leading to reactive lymph node enlargement. If such is the case a fine-needle biopsy may be required to rule out malignant spread.

Paget's disease (see page 87)

This important lesion appears as an erythematous, slightly scaly patch that may be pigmented, particularly on the nipple or the genital area, and is easily confused with dermatitis. Biopsy is essential for diagnosis. At the nipple the lesion is usually the result of malignant cells having migrated along the ducts from a breast carcinoma to lie in the skin.

Skin metastases

These are subcutaneous tumours that have seeded to the skin from another primary site. Often the primary tumour will already be known, otherwise the diagnosis is usually made on a biopsy and by a process of exclusion. It is important to exclude a curable primary site since it may be treatable, e.g. a lymphoma.

Treatment

Treatment is usually tailored to suit the situation, with the aim of eradicating the local disease and obtaining the best functional and cosmetic result.

Cure rates for non-melanomatous lesions are in the 90–99% range.

The main modes of treatment are surgery and/or radiotherapy to achieve local control.

Decisions are usually based on size, location, and aggressiveness of the tumour, as well as patient suitability for the procedure.

All tumours should have histological confirmation.

Surgery

Surgery offers a single procedure with a high cure rate.

The aim is to remove the lesion completely.

Frozen section examination can give immediate indication of marginal involvement.

If the margins are not clear, further excision must be carried out as soon as possible.

Healing may be by primary closure or secondary intention.

Radiotherapy

Radiotherapy, using an electron beam which has limited depth of penetration (the exact depth is dependent on the energy selected) can produce excellent results but needs to encompass the lesion and provide a margin of 10–15 mm surrounding it.

Usually multiple visits to the radiotherapy centre are needed for fractions of treatment.

A total dose of 45 Gy over 3 weeks in 3-Gy daily fractions would be a typical example.

Where biologically equivalent doses are given in shorter periods of time, the cosmetic result tends to be less satisfactory but such a compromise may be necessary in elderly patients or where long distance of travel is a problem.

Radiotherapy is a good choice for a patient who would not be keen or fit for surgery. It is less suitable where bone, cartilage, or tendons are involved because of the danger of radionecrosis.

Radiation is used in locations such as the eyelids and tip of the nose where surgical excision would involve extensive reconstruction. It is also useful where, following surgery, the histology shows tumour involvement of the surgical margins.

Melanoma

Incidence and mortality

In 2001 3,193 men and 4,128 women were diagnosed with melanoma in the UK.[1]

In 2003 934 men and 832 women died from melanoma in the UK.[2]

Melanoma is a neoplasm of the epidermal melanocyte whose primary function in the skin is to protect the body from excessive UV light.

Embryologically, melanocyte stem cells migrate from the neural crest in the fetus to the dermoepidermal junction and thus are found at non-cutaneous sites, e.g. mucous membranes, the eye, the central nervous system, and in lymph node capsules.

The melanocyte produces the brown-black pigment melanin from tyrosine via dehydroxyphenylalanine (DOPA). It has a protective effect, absorbing UV photons and reactive oxygen radicals produced by sunlight. The pathway is usually activated by UV radiation – a single exposure gives an increase in activity and size of existing melanocytes. Repeated exposure gives a further increase and eventually causes melanocyte numbers to increase. Racial differences are also pronounced, with the melanocytes of people with dark skins constantly producing large amounts of melanin.

The increase in melanomas is worldwide and probably reflects both increased incidence and greater awareness.

In contrast with BCC and SCC, young adults are affected as well as older age groups; 45% occur in the under 60s compared with 20% of other skin cancers.

Australia currently has the highest incidence of 17 cases per 100,000 per year. Studies, especially from Australia, have shown that prevention as well as early removal of thin skin lesions could significantly improve morbidity and mortality.

Risk factors

Skin types

People with fair skin, which tends to burn easily and tan poorly, are at greatest risk.

Severe sunburn, similar to radiation damage, appear to be cumulative, particularly in childhood.

It is hypothesized that melanoma is induced by acute sun exposure after a long period of non-exposure – the typical annual sunshine holiday that has become so popular over the last several decades.

By contrast, BCC and SCC are caused by the prolonged sun exposure seen in outdoor workers. Moles may arise in normal skin, in benign pigmented naevi, dysplastic naevi, or congenital melanocytic naevi. The last two are thought to be melanoma precursors.

Key Facts
Six skin types
Type 1 Always burns, never tans – white skin
Type 2 Initially burns, difficult tanning – white skin
Type 3 Rarely burns, easily tanned – white skin
Type 4 Never burns, always tans – white skin
Type 5 Brown skin
Type 6 Black skin

Moles (naevi) are thin lesions – no more than 1 mm in depth but with a diameter usually greater than 5 mm. They are rare in children. In adult women they occur mainly on the lower extremities and in men, mainly on the trunk.

Wherever they arise, although initially benign, they may undergo change to become established melanomas. This is often imperceptible. Most melanomas are thought to arise in a single transformed melanocyte.

The growth is initially in the horizontal axis at the basal lamina, known as the radial growth phase, and is non-metastatic. The duration of this phase varies with aggressiveness.

Eventually, dermal invasion ensues as the vertical growth phase takes over, leading to metastatic potential.

Genetics

Around 10% of patients with melanoma have a family history and an autosomal dominant gene with incomplete penetrance is likely.

Melanoma types

There are four types classified on growth patterns – superficial spreading, nodular, lentigo maligna, and acral lentiginous. Each has a unique natural history and features.

Superficial spreading or flat melanoma

- This is the commonest type (70%)

- It usually arises in a pre-existing naevus or dysplastic naevus and develops over 3–5 years

- The shape changes, the edge becoming irregular. The surface shows dark areas with colour variation and it becomes rough or even ulcerated

Nodular

- Whilst relatively rare (0–20%) this is the most aggressive

- It usually appears on normal skin and grows quickly – the volume may double in a few months

- It is typically blue/black, raised, or dome-shaped, and may look as if it is stuck on to the skin

Lentigo maligna melanoma (LMM)

- LMM (4–10% of melanomas) is usually seen on sun-exposed skin, especially on the face in the elderly and often in women

- It arises in a lentigo maligna (melanotic freckle) that has been present for a long time

- Since there is a prolonged radial phase, the lesions are generally flat, irregular in shape and large – up to 3 cm. The colour tends to be light to dark brown. The lesions develop over decades

Acral lentiginous melanoma (ALM)

- ALM (2–8% in white population but 35–60% in black population) occurs on the palms, soles, and subungal areas, and are usually large (> 3 cm diameter) and aggressive. The subungal lesions have a particularly bad reputation

- Early lesions may appear similar to LMM, but late lesions have a rapid vertical growth phase, giving ulceration and fungation

Clinical presentation

Clinically the lesions become larger, darker, and gradually develop an irregular outline. They also become thicker and gradually rise above the skin surface to become palpable.

Like an iceberg, a lesion palpable above the surface is likely to have a much larger component below. This invades into the dermis to gain early access to lymph vessels and the bloodstream, enabling systemic spread to other organs such as liver, lungs, brain, and bone.

The surface of a melanoma often has a mottled appearance.

The dark areas represent actively growing disease and are overproducing pigment.

Eventually bleeding from the surface may occur which is usually a late and sinister sign indicating dermal spread and vascular involvement.

Clinical diagnosis

Clinical diagnosis is based on appearance. No symptoms are expected with early lesions.

> **Key Facts**
>
> In the assessment of a pigmented lesion there are four clinical criteria which are suggestive of malignant melanoma:
>
> - A – Asymmetry of shape
> - B – Border notching (sharp and irregularly serrated)
> - C – Colour darkening (brown, black, or dark blue with uneven distribution)
> - D – Diameter enlargement (usually in excess of 7–9 mm)

Clinical examination should include examination for satellite lesions in the skin between the lesion and the regional lymph nodes, nodal enlargement, distant skin metastases, and hepatosplenomegaly.

Staging

This has advanced from the older anatomical staging of localized, regional, and disseminated to TNM staging which gives useful prognostic information to guide management of the patient with melanoma.

- The depth of invasion, thickness in millimetres, any ulceration, and growth patterns are all important features

- Where there is no lymph node involvement, thickness in millimetres and the presence of ulceration is of over-riding importance, correlating well with prognosis

- Clarke defined five levels of invasion (Fig 16.1). This system has been largely superceded by the Breslow thickness which is a better indicator of prognosis.

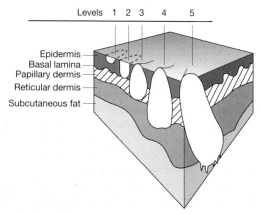

Fig. 16.1 Layers of the skin and Clark levels of tumour invasion.

Breslow made the depth measurement more accurate and reproducible by using an ocular micrometer.[3]

The vertical thickness in millimetres is measured from the epidermal granular layer (or the base of the lesion if there is ulceration) to the deepest melanoma cell identified.

TNM Staging

This is based primarily on Breslow thickness and ulceration on histology

T Stage

T1   Melanoma $\leq$ 1.0 mm thickness

T2   Melanoma 1.01-2 mm

T3   Melanoma 2.01-4 mm

T4   Melanoma > 4 mm

The T stage is subdivided into 'a' if no ulceration is present and 'b' if present. For T1 tumours only the presence of Clarke level 4 or 5 invasion is also classified as 'b'.

N Stage

N0   no nodes involved

N1   one node

N2   2-3 nodes or intra lymphatic regional metastases without nodal involvement

N3   4 or more nodes or intra lymphatic regional metastases with any nodal involvement

M stage

M1   distant metastases

Prognosis

Depth (thickness)

This is the most important factor affecting prognosis. The survival of patients with melanomas up to 0.75 mm is excellent.

Survival with thin lesions (< 1 mm) where the chance of metastasis is low, is good with 10-year survival in excess of 90%.

The deeper the lesion, the worse the outlook and as presentation is often late overall the 5-year survival is lower at 52% for men and 75% for women.

Ulceration

This is late in the history of the lesion and is a bad prognostic sign, especially if accompanied by bleeding, since it almost certainly means that there has been invasion into the deep layers of the dermis.

Sex

Women have a better prognosis than men, independent of other variables.

Age

Men aged over 50 years have the worst prognosis.

Site

Extremity sites (limbs) have a better prognosis than axial sites, e.g. head, neck, and trunk.

Type

A nodular melanoma or a nodular component within the lesion is more aggressive than other types.

Management

Surgery is the treatment of choice, first, to make a definitive diagnosis, and second, to remove the lesion.

Pigmented naevi are best excised *in toto*.

If histology confirms a diagnosis of melanoma of less than 2-mm depth and clear margins of clearance then the patient can be managed by being followed up.

If the margins are clear and it is thicker than 2 mm, or where the lesion is clinically an obvious melanoma, then a wider excision is carried out and the patient followed up.

Where the lesion is on the distal region of a digit, then amputation of the finger or toe is the best way to achieve adequate clearance.

Where cervical, axillary, or inguinal/iliac lymph nodes are enlarged, fine-needle aspiration of the nodes can be performed as well as investigation for evidence of widespread disease. If the nodes prove positive with no evidence of other disease, then radical dissection of the appropriate group is performed.

These are mutilating operations with considerable morbidity, usually best performed by plastic surgeons.

Lymphoscintigraphy is used to identify the first drainage or 'sentinel node(s)' within a group of nodes.

Sentinel node biopsy gives material for histology, immunohistochemical, or other detection such as molecular examination. If positive, the nodal metastases can then be treated by regional lymphadenectomy. The significance of sentinel node micrometastases is unclear (< 1 mm) and biopsy has not shown improved survival.

Local recurrences

These can be surgically excised. Depending on the size of the deficit, skin grafting may be required. A thorough search must be made for distant metastases.

Distant metastases

In spite of the apparent immunological phenomena associated with the disease, melanoma has been notoriously resistant to treatment with any other modality than surgery, despite sporadic dramatic results with interferon.

Adjuvant therapy

Patients with thick lesions or nodal involvement are at greater than 50% risk of recurrence, systemic disease, and death within 5 years, so adjuvant therapy should be considered as part of a good clinical trial where full assessment is being carried out.

This is the one cancer where historically there is more documented evidence of spontaneous regression than any other.

The regressions are thought to be due to the expression of antigens on the melanoma cells recognized as foreign by the immune system, which then mounts an attack against them. Many attempts have been made to try to enhance the host recognition and/or immunological response to melanoma cells.

Metastatic disease

Chemotherapy has modest impact on metastatic disease (response rate 20%) and the most commonly used agent is Dacarbazine (DTIC). Because of this, effort has concentrated on manipulation of the immune system. Interferon has been used for advanced disease and has produced regressions.

In another approach, vaccines made from partially purified melanoma antigens extracted from melanoma cell lines have been used.

Prevention

Because treatment of the established disease is so limited, primary prevention has assumed great importance. This has included use of sunscreen sprays, although sunscreens, whilst useful, should not be used as the sole protection.

References

1. http://info.cancerresearchuk.org/cancerstats/types/melanoma/incidence/
2. http://info.cancerresearchuk.org/cancerstats/types/melanoma/mortality/
3. Breslow A. Thickness, cross-sectional areas and depth of invasion in the prognosis of cutaneous melanoma. *Annals of Surgery* 1970, **172**, 902–908.

Chapter summary

- Skin cancer is the most common cancer diagnosed in the UK

- In the UK there is an annual 3% increase in rates of melanoma

- Most of the common cancers of the skin, apart from melanoma, are easily treated

- Pre-malignant lesions, *solar (actinic or senile) keratosis*

- Malignant lesions, *basal cell carcinoma, squamous cell carcinoma, Paget's disease*

- Cure rates for non-melanomatous lesions are in the 90–99% range

- Main modes of treatment are surgery and/or radiotherapy to achieve local control

- Radiotherapy is a good choice for a patient who would not be keen or fit for surgery, less suitable where bone, cartilage, or tendons are close because of the danger of radionecrosis

Melanoma

- Melanoma is a neoplasm of the epidermal melanocyte

- In contrast to basal cell carcinomas (BCC) and squamous cell carcinomas (SCC), young adults are affected as well as older age groups

- People with fair skin, which tends to burn easily, are at greatest risk

- Around 10% of patients with melanoma have a family history

Melanoma types

- *Superficial spreading or flat melanoma (70%)*

- *Nodular 10–20% (this is the most aggressive type)*

- *Lentigo maligna melanoma (LMM) 4–10%*

- *Acral lentiginous melanoma (ALM) (2–8% white population 35–60% black population)*

Assessment

- A – Asymmetry of shape

- B – Border notching (sharp and irregularly serrated)

- C – Colour darkening (brown, black, or dark blue with uneven distribution)

- D – Diameter enlargement

Staging

- Where there is no lymph node involvement, thickness in millimetres and presence of ulceration are of over-riding importance

Management

- Surgery is the treatment of choice

- Resistance to chemotherapy has been almost universal

- Immune therapies have been trialled

- Melanoma occasionally undergoes spontaneous regression

Patients with head and neck cancer

'In the face of such overwhelming statistical possibilities, hypochondria has always seemed to me to be the only rational position to take on life.'

John Diamond: *Because Cowards Get Cancer Too* (1998)

Background

- While head and neck cancers cause about 3% of all cancer deaths in the UK, the impact of these cancers on psychological, physical, and social functioning cannot be overstated
- Commoner in France, Italy, Poland, Thailand, and the Indian subcontinent
- Approximately 50% of patients are cured
- Mortality varies widely according to site, histology, stage at diagnosis, and degree of tumour differentiation; stage is the most important factor
- Early recurrence after primary treatment is a bad prognostic sign
- Many patients who survive 2 years without recurrence are likely to be cured
- Second primaries are very common, occurring in perhaps one in eight patients – the effects of these on prognosis are often dire
- There are two possible explanations for the high frequency of second primaries:
  - **Field change:** carcinogens that predispose to specific cancers (e.g. tobacco and alcohol) produce widespread epithelial changes which easily develop into malignancy
  - **Clonal expansion and migration** of malignant cells

Common aetiological factors

♦ Smoking and alcohol

♦ The effect of these two factors are synergistic, and they are the strongest factor in the causation of head and neck squamous cell carcinomas (HNSCC)

Tumours at particular sites also have local risk factors:

♦ Betel nut chewing, vitamin deficiencies for oral cancer

♦ Nickel, chromate, hardwood dusts for airways tumours

♦ Viruses: Epstein–Barr virus in nasopharyngeal carcinoma

♦ Iron deficiency: Patterson–Brown–Kelly syndrome (iron deficiency, koilonychia, glossitis, upper oesophageal web) associated with post-cricoid carcinoma

♦ Familial: increased risk of HNSCC if there are two or more first-degree relatives with HNSCC

Histology

Ninety per cent of head and neck tumours are **squamous cell carcinomas**.
This has a number of implications:

♦ Often moderately chemosensitive but not curable with chemotherapy

♦ Association with paraneoplastic hypercalcaemia

Less common tumours include adenocarcinomas, adenoid cystic carcinomas (salivary glands), anaplastic carcinomas, lymphomas, melanomas of the mucosa, and other rare tumours.

Staging

Squamous cell carcinoma (SCC) tends to progress from local disease, along lymph node levels in a stepwise manner, to distant disease occurring quite late. This allows radical treatment to be matched with treatment of the important lymph node groups, e.g. radical neck dissection.
Treatment has now improved so substantially that the cause of death is changing:

♦ Forty years ago only a small proportion of patients died of disseminated disease

♦ Now distant metastases are the cause of death in perhaps a third of patients and are found in many others[1]

♦ This has major implications for the issues being faced by patients with advanced head and neck cancer

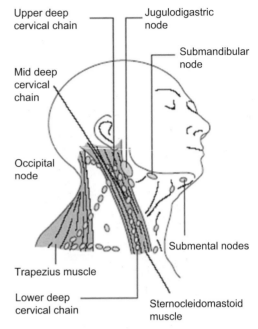

Fig. 17.1 Lymphatic drainage of head and neck.

Anatomical considerations

These are complex, for example, the posterior one-third, or base of tongue, is not mobile, and tumours involving this part are much more likely to spread to local lymph node stations at an earlier stage of the natural history. They also have more of a tendency to spread bilaterally, because of extensive lymphatic pathways which cross the midline.
The *maxillary sinus* is bounded by the following:

♦ Superiorly – floor of orbit and infra-orbital nerve

♦ Inferiorly – hard palate and alveolar process of the maxilla

♦ Medially – lateral wall of nasal cavity

♦ Anterolaterally – skin and fascia of cheek

The *nasopharynx* is formed into the shape of a truncated pyramid, being related superiorly to the sphenoid sinus and basal part of the occipital bone. The third and sixth cranial nerves run in the cavernous sinus in this region, thus extension of a nasopharyngeal tumour superiorly may cause cranial nerve palsies. The inferior boundary is the hard and soft palate, and posteriorly lies the retropharyngeal space containing nodes of Rouvière, which are directly anterior to the lateral processes of the atlas. In this region, the ninth and twelfth nerves run adjacent to the carotid sheath. The lateral walls are

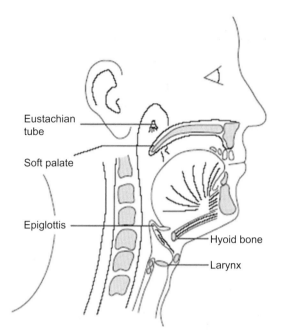

Fig. 17.2 Anatomical relationships of head and neck structures.

where the Eustachian tubes emerge, in the fossa of Rosenmueller, through which spread can occur into the parapharyngeal space and pterygoid muscles. '

Regions of the neck are subdivided into levels as follows:

♦ **Level I** – submental and submandibular triangles, bordered by the midline, anterior and posterior belly of the digastric muscle, mandible, and hyoid bone

♦ **Level II** – subdigastric area down to the carotid bifurcation, and from the jugular foramen to the posterior border of the sternocleidomastoid muscle. It also includes the upper posterior cervical triangle

♦ **Level III** – from the posterior border of the sternocleidomastoid to omohyoid muscle, stretching along the jugular vein between the carotid artery and its bifurcation

♦ **Level IV** – below the omohyoid muscle down to the level of the clavicle, anterior to the omohyoid and posterior to the carotid vessels

♦ **Level V** – from the posterior edge of sternocleidomastoid muscle to the trapezius muscle, and between the posterior belly of the omohyoid to the entrance of the spinal accessory nerve. This is the posterior cervical triangle

Examination

A full ear, nose, and throat (ENT) examination by a trained specialist is mandatory. Careful inspection of the oral cavity, buccal mucosa, and under the tongue, followed by palpation and indirect laryngoscopy can be performed in the outpatient department on the initial visit.

Inspection of the nasopharynx and external auditory meatus, and palpation for cervical or supraclavicular lymphadenopathy are also carried out. If indicated, direct laryngoscopy with inspection of the nasal cavity can also be performed, using local anaesthetic spray on the posterior pharyngeal wall. If a lesion is directly visualized, a detailed description of site, size, boundaries, and appearance needs to be documented and the lesion should be biopsied.

Tumours of the head and neck tend to grow as ulceration of the mucosal surface, with raised indurated edges. Palpation may be the best way of identifying the more subtle endophytic lesions, which tend to be more aggressive than the easily visible exophytic lesions. The cranial nerves should be systematically tested, including the infraorbital nerve if a tumour of the maxillary sinus is suspected.

The presence or absence of lymphadenopathy must be noted, and any palpable nodes should be categorized and measured. A simple sketch of the findings can be very helpful. It is important to take into account the dental appearance and nutritional status of the patient.

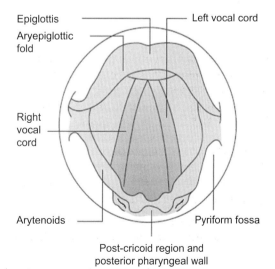

Fig. 17.3 Vocal cords.

TABLE 17.1 T staging for head and neck cancer

Site	T₁	T₂	T₃	T₄
Lip, oral cavity	≤ 2 cm	2–4 cm	> 4 cm	Invades adjacent structures
Oropharynx	≤ 2 cm	2–4 cm	> 4 cm	Invades bone, muscle, etc.
Larynx	Limited but mobile (a) One cord (b) Both cords	Extends to supra- or subglottis/impaired mobility	Cord fixation	Extends beyond larynx
Supra- and subglottis	Limited/mobile	Extends to glottis/mobile	Cord fixation	Extends beyond larynx
Hypopharynx	One subsite	> One subsite or adjacent site, without larynx fixation	With larynx fixation	Invades cartilage/neck, etc.
Nasopharynx	One subsite	> One subsite	Invades nose/ oropharynx	Invades skull/cranial nerves
Maxillary sinus	Antral mucosa	Infrastructure, hard palate, nose	Cheek, floor of orbit, ethmoid, posterior wall of sinus	Orbital contents and other adjacent structures
Salivary glands	≤ 2 cm (a) No extension (b) Extension	2–4 cm	> 4 cm	> 6 cm

Diagnosis

To make the definitive diagnosis, a biopsy is required, and often this will be done during an ENT examination under anaesthetic. If the patient presents with cervical lymphadenopathy and a primary site cannot be identified, fine-needle aspiration of a lymph node may need to be carried out, after a thorough ENT examination with blind biopsies of the nasopharynx. Computerized tomography scanning, or, more commonly, magnetic resonance imaging, can be particularly helpful for outlining the full extent of the primary tumour and also for identifying impalpable, but nonetheless enlarged, neck nodes. Positron emission tomography scanning is the latest tool to be employed in helping to assess the involvement of nodes.

Oral cavity tumours

Incidence and mortality

In 2001 2,868 men and 1,532 women were diagnosed with oral cancer in the UK.[2]

In 2003 1,018 men and 574 women died from oral cancer in the UK.[3]

TABLE 17.3 Incidence[3]

Site	Males	Females	Persons	M:F ratio
Lip (ICD10 C00)	245	114	359	2:1
Tongue (ICD10 C01–02)	784	455	1239	1.7:1
Mouth (ICD10 C03–06)	843	561	1404	1.5:1
Oropharynx (ICD10 C09–10)	532	185	717	2.9:1
Pyriform sinus (ICD10 C12)	207	44	251	4.7:1
Hypopharynx (ICD10 C13)	112	88	200	1.3:1
Other & ill-defined (ICD10 C14)	145	85	230	1.7:1
Oral cancer	2,868	1,532	4,400	1.9:1

ICD, International Classification of Diseases
Cancer Research UK, 2006, February, http://info.cancerresearchuk.org/cancerstats/types/oral/incidence/

TABLE 17.2 N staging for head and neck cancer

	N₁	N₂	N₃
All sites	Ipsilateral single ≤ 3 cm	(a) Ipsilateral single > 3–6 cm	> 6 cm
		(b) Ipsilateral multiple ≤ 6 cm	
		(c) Bilateral, contralateral ≤ 6 cm	

These are the most frequent head and neck cancers. They are usually well differentiated SCC, but tumours of minor salivary gland origin are also seen. Spread is predominantly local and to nodal groups in a stepwise manner. Larger tumours are more likely to have spread and have a poor prognosis. Midline tumours metastasize quickly to deeper cervical nodes and hence further afield. Anterior tongue carcinomas have a marked tendency to spread or recur despite adequate primary treatment.

Oral tumours can initially be treated with surgery, with or without radical neck dissection. Radiotherapy (external beam or brachytherapy) often gives equivalent results, with less functional impairment, but causes mucositis and xerostomia. Excellent dental care is essential with radiotherapy; dental sepsis can contribute to osteoradionecrosis. Relapse or tumours advanced at presentation require extensive surgery with major reconstruction. Late disease, or treatment, may cause dysarthria, dysphagia if the tongue is not mobile, and local ulceration and extension. A third of patients with tongue tumours develop multiple primaries.

Carcinomas of the sinuses

Paranasal sinus tumours (maxillary, ethmoid, frontal, sphenoid) are commonly well-differentiated SCC. They present late with local swelling, pain, ocular symptoms if the orbit is involved, and nasal or palatal extension with dental symptoms. Treatment is usually surgical with extensive reconstruction for cosmesis, followed by radiotherapy.

Salivary gland tumours

- Signs of malignancy
  - Facial palsy
  - Rapid growth
  - Hard infiltrating mass
- *Adenoid cystic carcinoma* is the commonest salivary cancer. It is slow growing and ulcerative. It is the tumour most likely to spread along perineural sheaths, leading to nerve palsies and neuropathic pain. It also infiltrates marrow cavities, so X-ray may miss its true extent
- *Adenocarcinomas* often have a relatively good prognosis because of their differentiation
- *SCCs* are more aggressive, cause pain, and metastasize early. They are more often metastatic than primary

- *Undifferentiated carcinomas* progress rapidly, and may mimic sarcomas
- A very small proportion of *pleomorphic adenomas* become malignant

Management is usually surgical, with radiotherapy for residual or recurrent disease, high-grade tumours or lymphomas. The facial nerve may be involved by tumour or sacrificed at operation.

Malignant melanoma

Malignant melanoma is commonest on the hard palate but also occurs on lower jaw, lips, tongue, or buccal mucosa. It is infiltrative and metastasizes early to lymph nodes. It often ulcerates and bleeds (see section on melanoma in Chapter 16).

Carcinoma of the larynx

Early disease presents with voice changes; late disease may also cause pain, stridor or dysphagia.

- **Glottic** (vocal cord) carcinoma is commonest. Nodal metastases occur late, because the cords have poor vascularity and lymphatic drainage, and the main determinant of prognosis is the T stage. Initial treatment consists of radiotherapy, which preserves function. Alternatively, surgery is equally successful but causes voice changes, although, as excision can be conservative since nodal spread occurs late, voice is often preserved. Combined radiosurgical or radiochemotherapeutic approaches are often needed in advanced disease
- **Supraglottic carcinoma** presents late, with vague dysphagia, referred ear pain, or cervical lymphadenopathy; hoarseness may signify involvement of the cords or adjacent structures. Progression is by local extension (to oropharynx, especially posterior third of tongue, hypopharynx, or glottis) or lymph node spread, because this region is richly vascular. Treatment is commonly by radical radiotherapy; surgery has to be radical (total laryngectomy[4]), but is unavoidable in certain settings, e.g. airway obstruction. Radical neck dissection may be warranted
- **Subglottic carcinomas** are rare but highly invasive. Pyriform fossa tumours behave like supraglottic tumours and have a poor prognosis. Postcricoid tumours may be associated with iron deficiency (Patterson–Brown–Kelly syndrome) and invade the hypopharynx circumferentially. Radiotherapy, radical surgery and chemotherapy have a role in management, depending on exact site and stage. Multidisciplinary assessment and management are essential

Carcinomas of the pharynx (comprising naso-, oro-, and hypo-pharynx)

These are usually squamous cell, though lymphomas are not unusual, especially if the tonsils or nasopharynx are involved.

◆ **Nasopharyngeal carcinomas** commonly present with nodal disease in the UK. They may also cause nasal obstruction, epistaxis, and otitis media from Eustachian tube obstruction. Lower cranial nerve palsies from base of skull extension, or third, fifth, and sixth nerve palsies from cavernous sinus invasion signify advanced disease. Growth into the posterior orbit also takes place. Some varieties of nasopharyngeal carcinoma have a tendency to haematogenous spread. Tumours are often anaplastic. Combined chemoradiotherapy is the treatment of choice. Unusually for head and neck cancers, irradiation of the neck is as effective as radical neck dissection. Radiotherapy requires meticulous planning to avoid damage to the upper spinal cord. Xerostomia is common from salivary gland irradiation. Chemotherapy is sometimes very effective. Late recurrences (over 2 years) can be retreated, even though, in principle, radiotherapy should not be given twice. Sometimes extended maxillectomy plus brachytherapy is used for recurrences

◆ **Oropharyngeal carcinomas** (posterior tongue, soft palate, fauces, tonsils, pharyngeal wall) frequently present late. They produce dysarthria, pain and risk of aspiration. Radical chemoradiotherapy is usual but extensive surgery with radical neck dissection followed by radiotherapy may be indicated in locally advanced disease

◆ **Hypopharyngeal carcinomas** are uncommon but have a poor prognosis as they occur in a silent area with late diagnosis. Aggressive treatment has, therefore, to be used judiciously

Principles of treatment

Head and neck tumours can be treated by surgery, radiotherapy or chemotherapy,[5] or by a combination of these modalities.

Surgical treatment operates on the principle that HNSCC spreads in an orderly manner through successive lymph node groups, so block dissection taking out tumour, nodes, and intervening lymphatics will control disease. The extent of disease-free margin which needs to be excised varies from tissue to tissue: if a tumour involves bone (e.g. mandible), muscle (e.g. tongue), or submucosal soft tissue and lymphatics (e.g. hypophar-

ynx), it requires wide excision even if the tumour itself is quite small. Furthermore, excision of structures invaded by tumour may be needed. Therefore major reconstruction is frequently required, e.g. skin, muscle, bone, or jejunal flaps, as well as the use of prostheses. This can preserve appearance and function to an impressive extent for many patients.

Salvage surgery for recurrence after radiotherapy usually has to be quite radical. This of course raises the question of the long-term benefit to the patient.[6] It is important to be radical when a substantial improvement in prognosis, function, or quality of life is likely but also to desist when the benefits are limited compared to the severe cost to the patient. This requires familiarity with the results of research into quality of life and body image, as well as a consideration of the interpersonal dimension.

The **treatment of neck nodes** is a central issue. Cervical nodal metastases are found in 40% of patients with HNSCC at diagnosis. As in lymph nodes from other tumours such as breast and melanoma, sentinel node biopsy is being used and the impact of micrometastases on treatment and prognosis is unclear.

Radiotherapy can sterilize small neck nodes or those from certain tumours (nasopharynx, thyroid) effectively, but surgery is needed in other cases.

Radical neck dissection removes all the nodes on that side, sternomastoid, internal jugular vein, and spinal accessory nerve, which supplies the trapezius and sternomastoid. This is effective but disabling, and more limited forms of neck dissection are now employed when appropriate,[7] often combined with radiotherapy or chemotherapy.

Radical radiotherapy often retains function better than surgery but causes other problems: mucositis, xerostomia, tissue fibrosis (which renders hazardous later salvage surgery in the face of recurrence), and occasionally damage to other structures, e.g. the spinal cord. Radiotherapy can be **external beam** or **brachytherapy** (radioactive implants, e.g. needles in the tongue). Fractionation into a larger number of small doses reduces adverse effects but very prolonged radiation regimens can reduce effectiveness. New technology (intensity modulated radiotherapy) reduces side effects such as xerostomia.

Palliative radiotherapy can address problems such as bone pain, dysphagia or stridor from paratracheal nodes, or bleeding or infection from fungating tumours.

Chemotherapy is potentially curative in some head and neck tumours, such as lymphomas, but not in HNSCC. The role of adjuvant or neoadjuvant chemotherapy is being explored.

Stop and Think

Why has prognosis not improved more in head and neck cancers?

The 5-year mortality rates from head and neck cancer have not significantly changed in the last 40 years despite advances in radiotherapy and surgical treatment. Nevertheless, they remain comparable to, or better than, common cancers such as breast and lung. Prognosis correlates closely with the stage of disease at presentation. Early cancers of the larynx, the commonest site in the head and neck, have a cure rate of 92–95%, contrasting with less than 10% cure rates for advanced tumours of the hypopharynx.

Management of patients with advanced head and neck cancer

There are many issues of symptom control in patients with advanced head and neck cancers. Issues include:

- Pain (often mixed nociceptive and neuropathic)
- Oral dysfunction with xerostomia, mucositis, and dental decay
- Interventions such as tracheostomy and gastrostomy
- Treatments of infections and fistulae
- Catastrophic bleeding may be a rare but devastating terminal event as when the carotid artery is eroded
- Poor body image may affect sexuality and social interactions
- Depression is common and risk of suicide is increased

Stop and Think

Carer support

It is crucial to assess and support the family, whoever the patient defines that to be. They see a loved one become severely disfigured and symptomatic, face communication problems and often frightening potential complications such as severe airways obstruction or bleeding. They need explanation, sensitively given information about the likely future, and special care for isolated relatives, young children, and those with severe health or other problems of their own.

CASE HISTORY

JD: Head and neck cancer

'My patient has been complaining of hoarseness for 4 weeks. Please advise.'

History

This 51-year-old politician, who has smoked 20 cigarettes per day since he was 15 years old, and who drinks 7 or 8 pints of beer per night at weekends, developed persistent hoarseness. He lives with his wife and has two married sons.

Examination

He appears well nourished, and is of good performance status. There is no cervical lymphadenopathy. On indirect laryngoscopy, there is a small lesion on the right vocal cord, extending to the anterior commissure but not onto the right vocal cord, nor into the supra- or subglottis. There is partial immobility of the right cord, but no fixation.

Investigations

Chest X-ray is normal. Biopsy confirmed well-differentiated invasive SCC.

Management

This man has a T_2N_0 SCC of the larynx and he should be offered radical radiotherapy.

Notes

Equivalent cure rates of 70% can be achieved with laryngectomy, or radical radiation therapy. For this man, the significant advantage of radiotherapy is voice preservation.

A CT scan is important to exclude a primary simultaneous lung carcinoma in these patients, who are at high risk.

Key Fact

Nociceptive pain is pain transmitted by an intact nervous system and is usually opioid sensitive.

Neuropathic pain is pain transmitted by a damaged nervous system characterised by pain with altered sensation.

Chapter summary

While head and neck cancers cause about 3% of all cancer deaths in the UK the impact of these cancers on psychological, physical, and social functioning cannot be overstated.

Common aetiological factors include:

- Smoking
- Alcohol

The effects of these two factors are synergistic, and they are the strongest factor in the causation of head and neck squamous cell carcinomas (HNSCC).

Histology: 90% of head and neck tumours are SCCs.

- Oral tumours can initially be treated with surgery, with or without radical neck dissection
- Radiotherapy (external beam or brachytherapy) often gives equivalent results, with less functional impairment, but causes mucositis and xerostomia

Paranasal sinus tumours (maxillary, ethmoid, frontal, sphenoid) are commonly well-differentiated SCCs. They present late with local swelling, pain, ocular symptoms if the orbit is involved and nasal or palatal extension with dental symptoms.

Carcinoma of the larynx, may present with voice changes, dysphagia, or stridor.

Carcinomas of the pharynx are usually squamous cell, though lymphomas are not unusual, especially if the tonsils or nasopharynx are involved.

- **Surgical treatment** operates on the principle that HNSCC spreads in an orderly manner through successive lymph node groups, so block dissection taking out tumour, nodes and intervening lymphatics will control disease
- The **treatment of neck nodes** is a central issue

References

1. Taneja C, *et al*. Changing patterns of failure of head and neck cancer. *Archives of Otolarygology – Head and Neck Surgery* 2002, **128**, 324–327.
2. http://info.cancerresearchuk.org/cancerstats/types/oral/incidence/
3. http://info.cancerresearchuk.org/cancerstats/types/oral/mortality/
4. Ward EC, *et al*. Swallowing outcomes following laryngectomy and pharyngolaryngectomy. *Archives of Otolarygology – Head and Neck Surgery* 2002, **128**, 181–186.
5. Gleich LL, *et al*. Therapeutic decision making in Stages III and IV head and neck squamous cell carcinoma. *Archives of Otolarygology – Head and Neck Surgery* 2003, **129**, 26–35.
6. Kowalski LP. Results of salvage treatment of the neck in patients with oral cancer. *Archives of Otolarygology – Head and Neck Surgery* 2002, **128**, 58–62.
7. Myers EN, Gastman BR. Neck dissection: an operation in evolution. *Archives of Otolarygology – Head and Neck Surgery* 2003, **129**, 14–25.

Patients with sarcomas

These **rare** malignant tumours of mesenchymal origin account for around 1% of all cancers but often occur in young people. In the past, treatment involved mutilating surgery and the prognosis was generally poor. Advances in surgery and chemotherapy mean that amputation is often avoided and survival has improved.

Sarcomas may arise almost anywhere in the body and typically present with a slow-growing mass and/or pain. They are difficult to diagnose because they are rare. Symptoms are often non-specific and they can be hard to distinguish from much more common benign tumours. X-ray abnormalities are easily missed, and histological diagnosis can be difficult, so specialist pathology and radiology are vital. Unfortunately, in many patients the diagnosis is delayed.

Classification

Classification of sarcomas is difficult; bone sarcomas can also occur in soft tissue (extra-osseous) sites and typically childhood tumours can occur in adults.

Definitive diagnosis requires biopsy. Fine-needle biopsies are difficult to interpret, but core biopsy at a site selected by the surgeon can be helpful. Incisional biopsy risks spreading tumour cells and local recurrence, and should be sited so that the area can be excised at definitive surgery.

There are many sub-types of sarcomas and their pathology is complex.

- Although some are named according to the tissues they resemble (e.g. leiomyosarcoma has features of smooth muscle), they may not arise from mature cells of those tissues

- The terminology has changed; malignant fibrous histiocytoma was a common diagnostic label 20 years ago but is now one of the less frequently diagnosed sarcomas

- Histological grade is important, predicting the risk of local relapse and/or distant metastasis

- In addition to immunohistochemistry, molecular techniques such as polymerase chain reaction, and fluorescence *in situ* hybridization can identify characteristic genetic changes. For example, 90% of Ewing's tumours are associated with rearrangements of the *EWS* gene on chromosome 22, most commonly with the *FLI-1* gene on chromosome 11

Four main clinical groups account for about 80% of patients with sarcoma and share many management principles:

- **Osteosarcoma and the Ewing's family of tumours**. Aggressive tumours mainly seen in children and teenagers that metastasize early. Treatment is complex, usually with pre-operative chemotherapy, followed by surgery, more chemotherapy and sometimes radiotherapy

- **Adult soft tissue sarcomas of limb, limb girdle, and trunk**. Commonest are leiomyosarcoma, liposarcoma, and synovial sarcoma. Surgery is the mainstay of treatment although high-grade tumours are usually also treated with radiotherapy. Chemotherapy is of modest benefit and usually reserved for palliation

- **Intra-abdominal sarcomas**. Surgery is the main treatment, but may not be possible because they are often in the retroperitoneum and present late. Local relapse is common and often not responsive to cytotoxic therapy. Gastrointestinal stromal tumour (GIST) is rare; treatment of relapsed or metastatic GIST has been revolutionized by targeted therapies

- **Rhabdomyosarcoma**. A childhood tumour that responds to intensive multi-modal therapy; the outlook is generally good with over 60% cured

Other sarcomas include *chondrosarcoma, giant cell tumours of bone, desmoid tumours*, and *Kaposi's sarcoma*.

Osteosarcoma and Ewing's family of tumours

Commonest malignant primary bone tumours are osteosarcomas; less frequently seen is the small round cell tumour, Ewing's sarcoma.

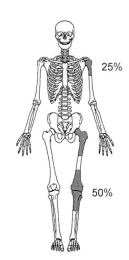

Fig. 18.1 Common sites of osteosarcoma.

Aetiology is unknown for most patients. Osteosarcoma may occur at sites of:

- Paget's disease of bone in older patients, where bone turnover rates may approximate those in the growing long bones of teenagers

- Prior radiotherapy, usually for an unrelated malignancy

Osteosarcoma

- 20% of primary bone cancers and 5% of childhood tumours

- Occur predominantly in adolescents and young adults (75% of tumours in patients < 20 years)

- A second peak in incidence seen in the elderly who are more likely to have Paget's disease, bone infarcts, or to have had prior radiotherapy

- Usually originates in the metaphyses of long bones, particularly the distal femur, proximal tibia, proximal femur, and humerus

Ewing's sarcoma

- 5–10% of bone cancers

- Most patients are 10–15 years old

- More evenly distributed in the skeleton than osteosarcoma, with a higher proportion of axial tumours

- Tumour permeates widely within the medullary cavity of the diaphysis and usually invades the periosteum

- Closely related to so-called primitive neuroectodermal tumours (PNET)

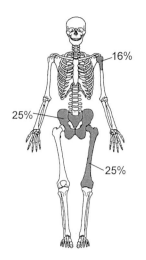

Fig. 18.2 Ewing's sarcoma: common sites of origin.

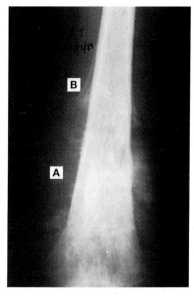

Fig. 18.3 Osteosarcoma: radiograph showing tumour of the lower femur with sun-ray spiculation (A) and bilateral periosteal elevation producing Codman's triangles (B).

Presentation

- Patients usually present with pain and abnormal X-ray. Pain is non-specific, especially in teenagers. Pain that comes at night or is persistent/progressive with no obvious cause should raise suspicion

- A slow-growing mass

- Occasionally a pathological fracture through the tumour

- Osteosarcomas may produce systemic symptoms that suggest advanced (metastatic) disease, which is present in 10–20% of patients at diagnosis, but can mimic osteomyelitis, creating diagnostic difficulties and delays

Investigations and staging

X-ray appearances of the affected bone include:

- An osteolytic (bone-destroying), expansile lesion that eventually breaches the cortex elevating the periosteum to give the characteristic picture of Codman's triangle

- Calcification in the surrounding soft tissue component. Spicules of bone forming at right angles to the long axis of the bone are called 'sun-ray spiculation'

A carefully planned biopsy is vital in making the diagnosis.

Once the diagnosis is confirmed, patients require:

- Computerized tomography (CT) scan of chest (for lung metastases)

- Magnetic resonance imaging (MRI) and bone scan (to assess extent of local disease/skip lesions in the same bone, or bone metastases)

- Bilateral bone marrow aspirates and trephines (Ewing's sarcoma only)

- Audiometry, renal, cardiac, and pulmonary function tests (as a baseline, to identify late effects of therapy)

Treatment

Historically, treatment with surgery alone, often amputation, was associated with a high rate of relapse and poor survival.

- Amputation can now be avoided in 70–90% of patients with extremity osteosarcoma because of both improvements in surgical technique and use of chemotherapy

- Whereas < 20% of patients with osteosarcoma and < 5% of patients with Ewing's sarcoma were cured prior to the use of effective chemotherapy, overall cure rates are now 50–80%

- The prognosis for patients with metastatic disease has improved but remains poor; patients with bone metastases rarely survive

Localized disease

- Pre-operative combination chemotherapy increases the number of patients in whom limb-sparing surgery is possible and allows histological assessment of response. Combination chemotherapy regimens incorporate some or all of the following drugs:

cisplatin, doxorubicin, methotrexate, etoposide, and ifosfamide

- Surgery in specialist centres using advanced endo-prosthetic engineering often allows tailor-made endo-prostheses to be surgically implanted, with limb salvage. Surgery is planned using MRI scans to assess the extent of local disease

- Adjuvant chemotherapy is used following surgery

- Radiotherapy is useful after surgery if residual local disease is present. In patients with Ewing's sarcoma, radiotherapy to the lungs may reduce the risk of relapse

TABLE 18.1 Principles of limb-sparing surgery
- Wide resection of involved bone. A 3–4-cm margin is taken beyond radiologically discernible abnormal bone
- A cuff of normal muscle tissue is removed in all directions
- Adjacent joint and capsule are resected
- No major neurovascular involvement
- All sites of previous biopsies and potentially contaminated tissue are resected *en bloc*
- Adequate soft tissue coverage
- Regional muscle transfers must be sufficient to allow adequate motor function

Treatment is intensive and long-term survival is common, so late side effects are important.

- Male patients are offered semen storage because of the risk of infertility; preservation of fertility for female patients is not yet routinely available

- Limb-sparing surgery in children may damage growth plates, leading to asymmetry as the normal limb grows. Modern endo-prosthetic implants that can be extended non-surgically may avoid the need for further surgery

- Radiotherapy is also associated with disruption of normal growth and an increased incidence of a second, radiation-induced malignancy

Advanced or metastatic disease

- For unresectable tumours, radiation in combination with chemotherapy gives a high rate of local control

- Pulmonary metastases are common but resection followed by chemotherapy may lead to long-term survival

- Chemotherapy may also be used as palliation

Key Facts
Good prognostic indicators for pulmonary metastases in osteosarcoma
- Fewer than five metastases
- Long disease-free interval since resection of the primary tumour
- Peripherally sited, easily resected lesions
- Unilateral pulmonary metastases

Adult soft tissue sarcoma of limb, limb girdle, and trunk

Soft tissue sarcomas are often highly treatable, given appropriate management within a multidisciplinary team in a specialized centre.

Histologically, soft tissue sarcomas are markedly heterogeneous and accurate diagnosis requires an adequate tissue sample in the hands of an experienced sarcoma pathologist. The commonest are leiomyosarcoma (features resembling smooth muscle); liposarcoma (fat), and synovial sarcoma (synovium); angiosarcoma (blood vessels), fibrosarcoma (fibrous tissue), lymphangisarcoma (lymphatics), and neurogenic sarcoma (nerves) also occur.

- Soft tissue sarcomas may originate in the lower limb (60%), trunk (15%), upper limb (20%), head and neck (5%)

- Any age group may be affected, but 40% arise in patients over the age of 55 years

- Benign tumours of the soft tissues are many times more common than soft tissue sarcomas (1,000 patients annually in the UK)

Aetiology

Most occur sporadically. There are a few well-recognized associations:

- Radiation

- Various rare inherited gene defect syndromes e.g. Li–Fraumeni (due to mutant p53), von Hippel–Lindau syndromes, and familial retinoblastoma. Gardner syndrome is associated with an increased incidence of *fibromatosis*. *Neurofibromas* and *neurofibrosarcomas* arise with increased frequency in neurofibromatosis type 1 (von Recklinghausen's disease); *malignant schwannomas* are also more common in this condition and in multiple endocrine neoplasia

- Chronic lymphoedema

Presentation and investigation

Usually present as a soft tissue mass.

Five clinical features should raise suspicion of malignancy: size > 5 cm; a tumour arising deep to the deep fascia; pain; a rapid increase in size, and recurrence at the site of a previous lesion.

Systemic symptoms suggest metastatic disease.

Further investigation will involve imaging of the mass, biopsy, and staging:

◆ Imaging (X-ray, CT scan or MRI)

  • To assess the size of the primary lesion and define local extent of disease in planning surgery and/or radiotherapy as indicated

  • Can guide percutaneous biopsy so that vital structures such as nerves and arteries are not damaged

◆ Biopsy with expert histological review is required to make the diagnosis. Tumour grade is an important prognostic factor

  • Fine-needle aspiration is non-invasive but has a low specificity and sensitivity for sarcomas

  • Open incisional biopsy has a poor reputation from bad planning of the incision and drain sites which can lead to tumour spread with very serious implications

  • Percutaneous core needle biopsy at a carefully selected site, often under ultrasound or CT guidance, is the method of choice

◆ Staging

  • The commonest site of metastasis is the lungs so CT scan of the chest is required, especially for high-grade tumours

Treatment

Combining conservative surgery with radiotherapy produces local control rates and overall survival that are equivalent to those produced by more radical procedures like amputation. Although local control rates can be as high as 90%, long-term outcomes remain poor because of the tendency for these tumours to metastasize (especially to the lungs).

Localized disease

◆ Complete surgical excision, including the track of any previous biopsy and with a wide margin of nor-

> **Key Facts**
>
> **Guidelines for pulmonary metastatectomy in sarcomas**
>
> ◆ Primary tumour is controlled
>
> ◆ No evidence of extrapulmonary metastases
>
> ◆ Metastases technically resectable
>
> ◆ General condition and respiratory status good enough for surgery

mal tissue, is the mainstay of therapy for localized soft tissue sarcomas

◆ Radiotherapy and wide local excision are equivalent in terms of local control to compartmental surgery. Radiotherapy has been used as sole treatment for patients unsuitable for surgery by virtue of frailty, tumour site, or patient choice

◆ Adjuvant chemotherapy may delay relapse but has not shown a clear survival benefit and is not routinely given

Metastatic/advanced disease

◆ In selected patients pulmonary metastatectomy may be curative, with 5-year survival of between 26% and 34%

◆ Many patients with metastatic or locally advanced, inoperable tumours benefit from palliative chemotherapy. Chemotherapy is based around doxorubicin and ifosfamide, either as a single agent or in combination; the newer drug trabectedin is also active. Tumour shrinkage is seen in 15–40% of patients; the higher response rates achieved with combination chemotherapy do not translate into a survival advantage and are associated with increased toxicity

Prognosis

A poor outcome for patients with soft tissue sarcomas is associated with:

◆ Size > 5 cm

◆ High-grade tumours

◆ Spread to regional lymph nodes or distant sites carry a worse prognosis

◆ Patients > 60 years old

Intra-abdominal sarcomas

Sarcoma can occur within the abdominal cavity or retroperitoneum. Presentation is often late as these tumours can become very large before causing symptoms.

Gastrointestinal tract sarcomas tend to metastasize to the liver first, whereas retroperitoneal sarcomas metastasize to the lungs.

- Where possible, the best treatment is complete surgical resection but this can be difficult and should be carried out in specialist units
- Radiotherapy is usually precluded by the toxicity of irradiating normal bowel and liver
- Chemotherapy is mostly reserved for palliation of metastatic or inoperable tumours

Gastrointestinal stromal tumours (GIST)

Rare, but the commonest mesenchymal gastrointestinal malignancy. GISTs may cause vague non-specific symptoms, or present acutely with haemorrhage or perforation. Appearances are characteristic at endoscopy. Histological diagnosis requires an experienced histopathologist. The cell surface receptor protein, KIT, is almost always overexpressed and can be detected by immunohistochemistry. Staging focuses on the liver as the main site of metastasis.

Treatment of metastatic GIST has been revolutionized by imatinib, which inhibits the intracellular tyrosine kinase domain of the mutated cKIT protein receptor that drives proliferation. While not curative, imatinib benefits about 80% of patients with metastatic GIST by improving quality of life and prolonging survival. This is a rapidly changing field with new agents emerging.

Rhabdomyosarcoma

- Rhabdomyosarcoma is the commonest soft tissue malignancy in children and infants with a median age at diagnosis of 4 years
- It is a curable disease in the majority who receive optimal therapy, with more than 60% alive 5 years after diagnosis
- The commonest sites of origin in order of frequency are the head and neck, the genitourinary tract, the extremities, and the thorax

There are three main histological subtypes: embryonal, alveolar, and pleomorphic. Embryonal rhabdomyosarcoma is the most common, typically arising in the orbit or genitourinary tract.

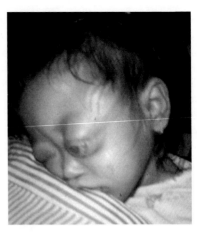

Fig. 18.4 Advanced rhabdomyosarcoma of the left orbit.

Treatment

Involves a multidisciplinary approach.

- All children should receive chemotherapy, the composition and duration of which depends on specialist assessment
- If possible, surgical resection is performed. The original extent of the tumour and the results of surgical resection govern decisions regarding radiotherapy
- In adults, these tumours carry a poorer outcome despite responding to paediatric chemotherapy regimens

Other sarcomas

Chondrosarcoma

Rare, malignant cartilaginous tumours.

- Second commonest matrix-producing bone tumour (after osteosarcoma)
- Typically seen in mid- to later life, and rare before the age of 30 years
- Men affected twice as commonly as women
- Associated with Paget's disease
- Arise most frequently in the central portion of the skeleton, particularly the shoulder, pelvis, and ribs
- Present as a slow-growing, painful, progressively enlarging mass

Presentation and investigations

- Usually present as slow-growing, painful, progressively enlarging masses

◆ Plain X-ray films show scalloping of the endosteum. The cortical appearance helps identify the likely grade; high-grade lesions cause cortical destruction and rapidly form a soft tissue mass, whereas low-grade tumours produce reactive cortical thickening

◆ Staging is as for osteosarcoma; the main sites of metastases are the lungs and bone

Treatment

Despite the low-grade nature of many of these tumours, complete surgical excision is important in avoiding locally recurrent disease, but can be challenging if limb salvage is also to be achieved.

Undifferentiated tumours are more sensitive to radiotherapy and chemotherapy.

Prognosis

◆ Most chondrosarcomas are well-differentiated grade I or II lesions which carry 5-year survival rates of approximately 90% and 80%, respectively

◆ Survival falls to around 40% for grade III tumours and is still lower for high-grade, undifferentiated disease

◆ Metastatic disease is rare in low-grade tumours, but may exceed 70% in higher-grade chondrosarcoma

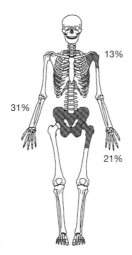

Fig. 18.5 Sites of chondrosarcoma.

> **Key Fact**
>
> **Grading** refers to the appearance of the cancer cells under the microscope and gives an idea of how quickly the cancer may develop. Low-grade chondrosarcoma means that the cancer cells look like normal cells, and they are usually slow-growing and less likely to spread. In high-grade tumours the cells look abnormal, are likely to grow more quickly and are more likely to spread. Chondrosarcomas are graded from I to III, with grade I being low-grade cancer and grade III high. Most chondrosarcomas are low-grade. Higher grade chondrosarcomas are more likely to recur and may spread to other parts of the body. Chondrosarcoma can occasionally develop into a more aggressive type of bone cancer known as dedifferentiated bone cancer.

Giant cell tumours of bone

◆ Giant cell tumours are uncommon, benign, but locally aggressive neoplasms

◆ They typically arise in early to middle adult life

◆ The majority develop around the knee but any bone may be affected

◆ Radiologically, they are large lytic lesions that are eccentric and often destroy overlying bone cortex

◆ A soft tissue mass may form surrounded by a shell of reactive bone

◆ Although appearing histologically benign, occasionally they may metastasize to the lungs

Management involves complete surgical excision; anything less is associated with a high rate of local recurrence.

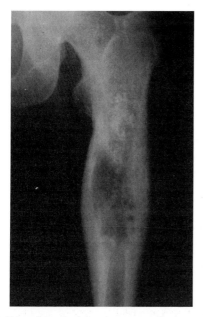

Fig. 18.6 Plain radiograph of chondrosarcoma affecting proximal left femur.

Kaposi's sarcoma (KS)

Four types of KS are recognized which, although of similar histopathological appearance, show different clinical features and course of disease.

- **Classic KS** – seen in elderly men of Italian/Eastern European Jewish ancestry; appears as single or multiple purple-red skin lesions on the lower limbs, especially around the ankles; slow, indolent course, but metastases finally develop. There is an increased risk of second malignancy, typically non-Hodgkin's lymphoma

- **African KS** – more common, endemic in the native population of equatorial Africa. Behaviour varies from relative indolence to aggressive, locally invasive disease. Shows a strong predilection for men, although of younger age than classic KS

Key Facts

Pre-AIDS Kaposi's sarcoma
First described in 1872 by Moritz Kaposi, an Austro-Hungarian dermatologist, this dermal tumour warrants specific mention because of its association with AIDS.
   Prior to the HIV epidemic KS was rare.

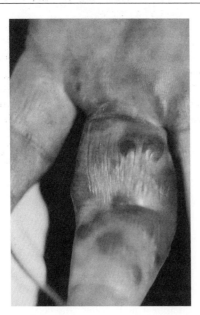

Fig. 18.7 Kaposi's sarcoma.

- **Immunosuppressant therapy KS** – particularly in patients with transplanted organs. Discontinuation or modulation of immunosuppressant treatment may produce disease regression and should always be considered in this setting

- **Epidemic KS** – fulminant and often widely disseminated form of the disease. First described in young homosexual and bisexual men in 1981. The presence of human herpesvirus 8 has been clearly linked to KS but the virus has not been shown to transform cells, which would more strongly suggest causation. The incidence of KS within the AIDS population is linked to the mode of disease acquisition. Heterosexual and intravenous drug users with HIV have a much lower risk of KS than those with homosexually acquired disease. The incidence of KS in AIDS patients is falling. The lesions may affect skin, oral mucosa, lymph nodes, or visceral organs although typically opportunistic infection is the cause of death

Homosexual men without any evidence of HIV infection are also at increased risk of KS, although this form of the disease is more typically indolent and affects the genitalia and extremities.

Treatment

Depends on the type and extent of disease.

- Single or small numbers of cutaneous lesions (non-AIDS-related) may best be treated with low-dose local radiotherapy. Intra-lesional chemotherapy with such agents as vinblastine can also be effective. Sometimes simple cosmetic camouflage may be sufficient, but this often does not conceal the full thickness of the lesion or its nodularity

- AIDS-related KS is usually controlled by effective anti-viral therapy for the HIV infection and will usually resolve spontaneously while the viral load is kept under control. Florid AIDS KS is now mainly seen as part of late-presenting untreated AIDS or in the terminal phase when drug resistance has developed

- Severe oro-cutaneous or symptomatic visceral disease requires systemic therapy and chemotherapy with low-dose liposomal doxorubicin. This is usually highly effective but often only controls the disease temporarily

Desmoid tumours

- Also known as aggressive fibromatoses

- Aetiology is unclear, but found in association with some genetic diseases such as Gardner's syndrome

- Although they do not metastasize, they may be locally destructive and progress relentlessly, possibly with fatal consequences, depending on their location

- Patients with unresectable lesions, or who are unfit for or decline surgery, may be treated with radiotherapy

- Local control of the tumour is possible in most cases though local recurrence remains a possibility

- The majority will be cured with radiotherapy

CASE HISTORY

RO: Boy with sarcoma

Four years ago a 13-year-old (RO) boy presented to his GP with a 2-month history of pain in the left knee. The pain had been increasing, was particularly noticeable at night, and the boy had begun to limp. The attendance at the GP was precipitated when swelling developed just proximal to the knee joint.

Plain radiographs of the lower femur showed a large, poorly delineated sclerotic and destructive lesion in the metaphyseal region. The lesion had breached the cortex and the periosteum was elevated, giving rise to the classical appearance of Codman's triangle. Bone spicules were visible at right angles to the long axis of the femur. CT and MRI scanning showed a destructive tumour without any evidence of neurovascular invasion.

A core needle biopsy confirmed the presence of osteosarcoma. Staging CT scans of the lungs showed no evidence of lung metastases and an isotope bone scan showed only the tumour at the lower end of the femur; there were no skip lesions or distant bone metastases. An echocardiograph was normal.

Discussion at a specialist multidisciplinary meeting reviewed the diagnosis and management options, and established a treatment plan.

Treatment commenced with two cycles of chemotherapy with cisplatin and doxorubicin. This was well tolerated with the exception of a lower respiratory tract infection associated with mild neutropenia, midway through the second cycle. This responded quickly to broad-spectrum antibiotics.

Repeat MRI scanning after two cycles of chemotherapy showed significant reduction in tumour size and changes in the signal, in keeping with marked tumour necrosis. Resection of the lower femur, upper tibia, and fibula was performed 5 weeks after the second cycle of chemotherapy and an endo-prosthesis and artificial joint were inserted. Histopathology confirmed almost 95% tumour necrosis with little viable osteosarcoma remaining. The margins of excision were all clear of disease.

A further four cycles of cisplatin and doxorubicin were delivered.

RO remained well until 2 years later, when a routine chest radiograph revealed a solitary lung metastasis. CT scanning confirmed the solitary nature of the lesion; examination and radiological imaging of the site of previous surgery showed no evidence of locally recurrent tumour. An isotope bone scan was unremarkable. The metastatic lesion was surgically resected. RO, now 18 years old, remains alive and well and free of disease.

Chapter summary

- **Malignant primary bone and soft tissue Tumours**
  – These are rare and the aetiology of most malignant primary bone tumours is unknown

Clinical presentation

- Local pain
- Development of a slow-growing mass
- Occasionally a pathological fracture through an involved bone
- Diagnosis requires careful imaging and expert pathology review

Management

- Most patients will require treatment involving a combination of surgery and chemotherapy
- The principles of limb-sparing sarcoma surgery are now well established in specialized centres
- The risk of local recurrences is increased in three situations:
  - Post-operative residual microscopic disease
  - Pre-operative pathological fracture
  - Open biopsy tracks which cannot be adequately excised at surgery
- Metastectomy is appropriate in selected patients
- Metastatic disease may respond to palliative chemotherapy or radiotherapy

Osteosarcoma and Ewing's Sarcoma

Osteosarcoma is a bone tumour occurring predominantly in adolescents and young adults

- It accounts for 20% of primary bone cancers and 5% of childhood tumours. Seventy-five per cent of tumours are seen in patients younger than 20 years
- Between 60 and 80% arise around the knee in younger patients
- Primary malignant round cell tumour of bone closely related to a group of tumours known as primitive neuroectodermal tumours (PNET)
- 6–10% of primary malignant bone tumours
- Most patients are between 10 and 15 years

Adult Soft tissue sarcomas

- Soft tissue sarcomas are rare (1,000 patients annually in the UK) but can occur at any age.

Intra-abdominal sarcomas

- Often present late
- GIST is a subtype that often responds to the tyrosine kinase inhibitor imatinib

Rhabdomyosarcomas

- Rhabdomyosarcomas represent the commonest soft tissue malignancy in children and infants with a median age at diagnosis of 4 years

Other Sarcomas

- Chondrosarcomas are malignant tumours of cartilage
- Second commonest matrix-producing bone tumour
- Typically arise in mid- to later life and rare before the age of 30 years

Kaposi's Sarcoma

- Four types of Kaposi's sarcoma are recognized which, although of similar histopathological appearance, show different clinical features and course of disease:
  - **Classic KS**
  - **African KS**
  - **Immunosuppressant therapy KS**
  - **Epidemic KS**

Giant cell tumours

- Giant cell tumours are uncommon, benign, but locally aggressive neoplasms
- They typically arise from mesenchymal tissue

Desmoid Tumours

- These uncommon tumours are benign but locally aggressive with a propensity for local recurrence following apparently complete resection

Patients with major cancer emergencies

Definition

An oncological emergency is defined as a situation arising in the cancer patient, related either to the cancer itself or its treatment, for which early diagnosis and treatment are necessary to prevent major morbidity or mortality.

Optimal outcomes in these patients rely on recognition of early symptoms and signs, and institution of the appropriate therapy. Avoidance of undue morbidity and mortality is particularly important for patients in whom further treatment may significantly prolong or improve the quality of life.

This chapter deals with five of the most significant oncological emergencies related to both cancer and to cancer treatment:

- Sepsis in the neutropenic patient
- Spinal cord compression
- Superior vena caval obstruction (SVCO)
- Haemorrhage
- Hypercalcaemia

General emergency awareness

It is important to have a clear understanding of the management of emergencies in oncology. Clear thinking is crucial in handling an emergency and a sense of calm authority can provide a source of decisiveness to patient and family and transform a crisis situation.

All health care professionals involved with the care of patients with cancer must be aware of the emergency situations which require a prompt response.

Optimal management of oncological emergencies requires:

◆ Prompt recognition of the clinical syndrome

◆ Knowledge of the cancer's natural history

◆ Appreciation of the aims of treatment

◆ Awareness of the side effects of the treatment

◆ Prompt initiation of appropriate management

Sepsis in the neutropenic patient

All health care professionals in contact with cancer patients need to be aware of the risks of a lowered immune response, specifically neutropenia. Typically this happens in the second week after chemotherapy,

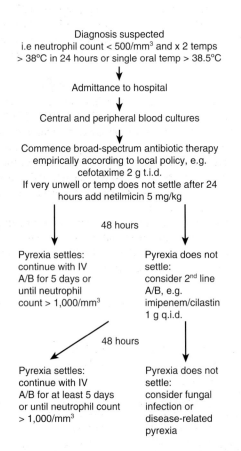

Antibiotics until neutrophil count > 1,000/mm³

Fig. 19.1 Example of a neutropenic sepsis protocol – Treatment options should be discussed with the local bacteriologist, as antibiotic regimens and neutropenic sepsis protocols will vary across the country, and should include consideration of antibacterial, fungal, and viral therapy. A/B = antibiotics.

the 'nadir' period, although it can occur earlier or later. Patients on chemotherapy should be instructed to contact the oncology unit urgently if they become unwell and have symptoms compatible with sepsis.

Manifestation of sepsis in a patient who is undergoing oncological treatment can be minimal, and there should be a high index of suspicion. The routine signs of a raised temperature, a fast pulse, and sweating may be absent. Without such vigilance, patients may suddenly deteriorate and become septicaemic which, for a significant proportion, will be fatal.

Management

◆ Awareness of the seriousness of this risk for patients who have recently undergone oncological treatments

◆ Prompt checking of a white cell count to confirm the risk in susceptible patients about whom you are concerned

◆ Admission of all patients with neutropenic sepsis for intravenous antibiotics can be given and appropriate monitoring in a specialized unit

◆ Empirical treatment of the ill neutropenic patient while blood culture results are awaited, including intravenous fluids and antibiotics

◆ Granulocyte colony-stimulating factor can expedite recovery of neutrophils

Spinal cord compression

Spinal cord compression occurs in 3–5% of patients with cancer, and 10% of patients with spinal metastases develop cord compression,[1] the frequency being highest in patients with multiple myeloma and cancers of the prostate, breast, and bronchus.

It is important for all health professionals to have a high index of suspicion for possible spinal cord

Key Facts
Symptoms and signs of spinal cord compression
◆ Back pain 90%
◆ Weak legs
◆ Increased reflexes
◆ Sensory level
◆ Urinary hesitancy or retention
◆ Constipation

compression because of the catastrophic consequences of a delay in diagnosis.

◆ Back pain (especially if it radiates around the chest like a band), a sensation of weakness in the legs and often vague sensory symptoms may be **early manifestations**

◆ Profound weakness, a sensory 'level', and sphincter disturbance, are all relatively **late features**, by when the outcome is poor and the compression is much less likely to be reversible

◆ 80% of cases are caused by extradural deposits as a result of direct extension from the vertebral body into the anterior epidural space. Lesions above L1 (lower end of spinal cord) will produce upper motor neurone signs and often a sensory level, whereas lesions below L1 will produce lower motor neurone signs and perianal numbness (cauda equina syndrome)

The site of compression is:

◆ Thoracic in 70%

◆ Lumbosacral 20%

◆ Cervical 10%

◆ Multiple sites 20%

The keys to diagnosing spinal cord compression include:

◆ Having a high index of suspicion in patients with spinal metastases, particularly in those with multiple myeloma, breast, lung, or prostate cancer

◆ Taking patients' complaints about back pain, difficulty in walking, and difficulty in passing urine seriously

Patient assessment

If spinal cord compression is suspected two questions need to be answered urgently:

◆ **Does this patient have a reasonable likelihood of having spinal cord compression?** Even the most skilled clinician has difficulty in diagnosing spinal cord compression with absolute certainty. Often by the time clinical signs are 'classical' it is 'too late'. Once the compression has fully developed treatment outcome is very poor. Thus if intervention to prevent paralysis and incontinence is to be effective, spinal cord compression needs to be diagnosed early

◆ **Would this patient benefit from emergency investigation and treatment?** Once the possibility of spinal cord compression has been raised, the patient may now be committed to a course of management that will include urgent transfer to a specialized unit

---

Key Fact

Urgent referral

Where suspicion of spinal cord compression is high, it is quickest to involve the oncological team who have been managing the patient, who will be able to coordinate the necessary scan and appropriate treatment rapidly.

---

where a magnetic resonance imaging scan can be carried out and radiotherapy or surgery can be performed. Deciding whether this course of treatment is appropriate for a particular patient involves an overall assessment

If the patient is still walking, emergency treatment gives a 1 in 3 chance of regaining leg strength and **treatment should be started immediately with dexamethasone 16 mg daily orally** while arrangements are made for **urgent transfer** to an oncology centre.

Prognosis

Overall, 30% of patients with spinal cord compression may survive for 1 year. Function will be retained in 70% of patients who were ambulant prior to treatment but will return in only 5% of those who were paraplegic at the outset. Return of motor function is better in those with an incomplete block and particularly with partial lesions of the cauda equina. Loss of sphincter function is a bad prognostic sign.

In practice, many patients with an established diagnosis are relatively unwell and have multiple metastases, and will be referred for radiotherapy, achieving similar results to those of surgery.

TABLE 19.1 Indications for surgical decompression and radiotherapy

Indications for surgical decompression	Indications for radiotherapy
1) Uncertain cause – to obtain histology	1) Radiosensitive tumour
2) Radioresistant tumour, e.g. melanoma, sarcoma	2) Several levels of compression
3) Unstable spine	3) Unfit for major surgery
4) Previous radiotherapy	4) Patient choice
5) Major structural compression	
6) Cervical cord lesion	
7) Solitary vertebral metastasis	

Management of patients with residual paraplegia/quadriplegia

Such patients provide great challenges to the multi-disciplinary team. These challenges include:

- Mobility management, within the limits considered safe for the compromised spinal cord

- Pain control

- Skin care in a patient confined to bed

- Bowel interventions

- Urinary system management

- Psychosocial support

- Occupational and physiotherapy assessments

- Provision of equipment and advice on environmental changes

- Passive movements to maintain joint range

- Teaching carers on how to correctly undertake handling activities to maximize patient function and safety and allow for the possibility of care at home if appropriate

Superior vena caval obstruction (SVCO)

SVCO is due to compression or invasion of the SVC by mediastinal lymph nodes, thrombus, or tumour in the region of the right main bronchus.

It is caused most commonly by carcinoma of the bronchus (75%) or lymphomas (15%). Cancers of the breast, colon, oesophagus, and testis account for the remaining 10%. Symptoms are those of venous hypertension and include breathlessness (laryngeal oedema), headache (cerebral oedema), visual changes, dizziness, and swelling of the face, neck, and arms.

Signs include engorged conjunctivae, peri-orbital oedema, non-pulsatile dilated neck veins, and dilated collateral veins (chest and arms).

Without treatment, SVCO can progress over several days to death.

Prognosis is poor in a patient presenting with advanced SVCO unless the primary tumour is responsive to radiotherapy or chemotherapy.

Management – emergency treatment

For advanced, acute SVCO:

- Sit patient upright and give 60% oxygen

Key Facts

The **superior vena cava (SVC)** lies on the right side of the upper mediastinum, and is closely related to the aorta, right main bronchus, right pulmonary artery, and trachea.

It drains the jugular and subclavian veins, which supply the head, neck and arms.

It is susceptible to compression because of the low pressure within it, and also because of its location within the relatively rigid bony thorax.

Causes of SVCO may be classified as follows:

- **Benign:** e.g. goitre, mediastinal fibrosis

- **Malignant:** may be the result of tumour compressing or invading the SVC

- **Thrombosis:** as a primary event, this is usually related to the presence of an indwelling catheter for venous access; as a secondary event, this is usually due to sluggish blood flow related to obstruction

---

- Maintain calmness among staff (and patient/relatives) and consider low-dose midazolam subcutaneously to reduce patient anxiety, and thus improve the efficiency of respiration

- Dexamethasone 16 mg (oral or intravenous)

- Furosemide 40 mg (oral or intravenous)

- Emergency radiotherapy (or chemotherapy for chemosensitive tumours such as small cell carcinoma of bronchus, lymphoma, or testicular cancer) can be given with steroid cover (e.g. dexamethasone 16 mg daily)

- Survival may be prolonged for several months by treatment but recurrence may be more difficult to control

- Stents are increasingly used as a palliative measure. Intraluminal stents, inserted via the femoral vein, can also be considered in consultation with the local oncologist and radiologist and may provide rapid relief

Haemorrhage

Haemorrhage may be directly related to the underlying tumour or caused by treatment such as steroids or non-steroidal anti-inflammatory drugs resulting in gastric/duodenal erosion and haematemesis.

A generalized clotting deficiency, seen in haematological malignancies and thrombocytopenia, hepatic insufficiency or anticoagulation with warfarin, are also potential contributory factors in patients with cancer.

Treatments for non-acute haemorrhage

Treatments include:

- ◆ Oncological
- ◆ Systemic
- ◆ Local measures

Oncological

- ◆ Palliative radiotherapy is useful for superficial tumours and those of the bronchus and genito-urinary tract

Systemic

- ◆ If radiotherapy is not appropriate, coagulation should be enhanced with oral tranexamic acid 1 g t.d.s., but caution is necessary with haematuria since clots may form in the bladder resulting in further retention problems. The risks of encouraging hypercoagulation need to be considered carefully in patients with a history of a stroke or ischaemic heart disease

Local measures

- ◆ Topical tranexamic acid or adrenalin (1 : 1000) soaks may be useful
- ◆ Sucralfate may stop stomach mucosal bleeding although it will inhibit the absorption of a proton pump inhibitor such as lansoprazole

Acute haemorrhage

Erosion of a major artery can cause **acute haemorrhage** which may be a rapidly terminal event. It may be possible to anticipate such an occurrence and appropriate medication and a dark-coloured blanket to reduce the visual impact should be readily available.

Relatives or others who witness such an event will need a great deal of support.

If the haemorrhage is not immediately fatal such as with a haematemesis or bleeding from the rectum, vagina or superficially ulcerated wound, the aim of treatment is local control if possible and sedation of a shocked, frightened patient. Rectal or sublingual diazepam (or midazolam 5–10 mg subcutaneously or buccally) act quickly.

It may be appropriate to have emergency medication in the home to sedate the acutely bleeding patient, but such a strategy needs discussion with the family, carers, and the patient's local GP, and needs to be documented clearly. It is sometimes appropriate to treat haemorrhage with angiography and embolization, and even with surgery.

Hypercalcaemia

Hypercalcaemia occurs as a result of increased osteoclastic activity, which releases calcium from bone, in addition to a decrease in excretion of urinary calcium.

This is attributed to locally active substances produced by bone metastases or by factors such as ectopic parathyroid hormone-related protein or cytokines, and occurs in 10% of patients with cancer. The tumours most commonly associated with hypercalcaemia include squamous cell carcinoma of the bronchus, carcinoma of the breast and prostate, multiple myeloma, and other squamous cell tumours.

A corrected plasma calcium concentration above 2.6 mmol/l defines hypercalcaemia.

It is often mild and asymptomatic, and significant symptoms usually only develop with levels above 3.0 mmol/l. Levels which rise quickly to 4.0 mmol/l and above will cause death in a few days if left untreated. Eighty per cent of patients with cancer-related hypercalcaemia survive less than 1 year.

Symptoms include drowsiness, confusion, nausea, vomiting, thirst, polyuria, weakness, and constipation.

Stop and Think

When is too much information inappropriate?
The health care team need to balance the anxiety of alerting the family to the possibility of an acute bleed with the likelihood of such an event occurring and the need for the family to be prepared.

If the patient chooses to be looked after at home the issues surrounding managing acute haemorrhage need to be considered with the local team.

Key Fact

Corrected calcium
It is important to correct the calcium level if the albumin is reduced.

Add 0.02 mmol/l for every g/dl of albumin below 40 (which is the standard level) i.e. a serum calcium of 2.2 mmol/l with an albumin of 30 gives a corrected calcium of 2.4 mmol/l.

Management

Treatment is only necessary if there are symptoms, or a high likelihood of symptoms developing, and may be unnecessary if the patient is very near to death.

Fluid replacement and bisphosphonates

Intravenous hydration is the mainstay of acute therapy for severe or symptomatic hypercalcaemia.[2] Bisphosphonates intravenously can then be given. These drugs inhibit osteoclast activity and thereby inhibit bone resorption. They are given intravenously, and plasma calcium levels should start to fall after 48 hours and fall progressively for up to 6 days. Depending on the preparation, calcium levels can be controlled for 2–5 weeks by a single infusion. Such patients can have their calcium levels controlled by regular bisphosphonates given either intravenously or orally.

References

1. Kaye P. *Decision making in palliative care*. Northampton: EPL Publications, 1999: 183.
2. Bower M, Cox S. Endocrine and metabolic complications of advanced cancer. In: Doyle DH, *et al*, eds. *Textbook of palliative medicine*. 3rd edn. Oxford: O.U.P., 2004: 687–702.

Index

Note: page numbers in *italics* refer to figures, tables, and boxes.